Praise for *The Tyranny of Thinness*

"Bold, intimate, and philosophically rich, *The Tyranny of Thinness* is an essential guide to how the thinness ideal got its claws in us, and how to get free. Leboeuf conveys the pain of eating disorders, the punitive beauty norms of modeling, and the self-care that facilitated her recovery with lucidity and verve."

—KATE MANNE, professor of philosophy at Cornell University and author of *Unshrinking: How to Face Fatphobia* and *Down Girl: The Logic of Misogyny*

"If you think philosophy has no relevance to life, read this book. If you think there's nothing new to say about eating disorders, you'll find, with delight, that you're wrong. If you are a teacher trying to bridge the gap between 'theory' and lived experience, put this book on your syllabus. If you struggle with eating and body image issues and are tired of the same prescriptions—both from medical professionals and from the culture—that have been offered to you so far, I promise you will finish this book feeling refreshed and hopeful. I did!"

—SUSAN BORDO, professor of gender and women's studies and Otis A. Singletary Chair in the Humanities at the University of Kentucky and author of *Unbearable Weight: Feminism, Western Culture, and the Body*

"*The Tyranny of Thinness* is a clear and deeply humane account of why being slim still carries such power and how we might loosen its grip. Leboeuf's approach is philosophically serious and tender. Moving effortlessly between memoir and critique, she offers ideas and practices that can help us see ourselves and others more lovingly. Vivid, nuanced, and gently radical, this timely and optimistic book is exactly the kind of guide we all need to revalue our values about bodies, beauty, and freedom."

—SKYE CLEARY, PhD, MBA, philosopher and author of *How to Be Authentic* and *Existentialism and Romantic Love* and coeditor of *How to Live a Good Life*

"*The Tyranny of Thinness* offers an engaging look at the pressures cis women and girls face around body image and dieting. Leboeuf weaves personal stories with cultural critique to explore how society shapes our relationship with food and with ourselves. You'll find historical context and feminist analysis alongside practical tips for building a healthier relationship with your body. It's a valuable guide to breaking free from our culture's obsession with thinness."

—CAROL HAY, professor and department chair in the Department of Philosophy at the University of Massachusetts Lowell and author of *Think Like a Feminist*

"Part memoir, part self-help, and part philosophy, *The Tyranny of Thinness* confronts the reader with the reality of the overwhelming pressures to be thin in contemporary society. Pressures that are deep-rooted, almost impossible to resist, and yet often normalized. Leboeuf explains how the thin ideal has captured our minds and bodies, shares her experience of living with, recognizing, and overcoming anorexia, and offers solutions. She suggests practices to help us live from the inside out, including self-care, reclaiming pleasure, and communal resistance. This searingly honest book is a must-read for academics working on beauty, those suffering from and recovering from eating disorders, and anyone who has ever worried about their weight."

—HEATHER WIDDOWS, professor of philosophy at the University of Warwick and author of *Perfect Me: Beauty as an Ethical Ideal*

the tyranny of thinness

UNDERSTANDING AND RESISTING THE PRESSURE TO BE SKINNY

céline leboeuf, phd

North Atlantic Books
Huichin, unceded Ohlone land
Berkeley, California

North Atlantic Books
An educational nonprofit organization
Huichin, unceded Ohlone land
2526 Martin Luther King Jr Way
Berkeley, CA 94704 USA
www.northatlanticbooks.com

Cover design by Amanda Weiss
Interior design by Happenstance Type-O-Rama

Acquisitions editor: Shayna Keyles • Production editor: Maureen Forys, Happenstance Type-O-Rama • Copyeditor: Matthew Hoover
Proofreader: Christopher Church • Indexer: Rachel Kuhn

North Atlantic Books's publications are distributed to the US trade and internationally by Penguin Random House Publisher Services. For further information, visit our website at www.northatlanticbooks.com.

The authorized representative in the EU for product safety and compliance is Eucomply OÜ, Pärnu mnt 139b-14, 11317 Tallinn, Estonia, hello@eucompliancepartner.com, +33757690241.

Library of Congress Cataloging-in-Publication Data
Names: Leboeuf, Céline author
Title: The tyranny of thinness : understanding and resisting the pressure to be skinny / Céline Leboeuf.
Description: Berkeley, CA : North Atlantic Books, [2026] | Includes bibliographical references and index. | Summary: "This book serves as a guide to self-love and body trust, utilizing concepts from feminist philosophy as a path to reevaluating and redefining our contemporary notions of body acceptance" — Provided by publisher.
Identifiers: LCCN 2026001313 (print) | LCCN 2026001314 (ebook) | ISBN 9798889844068 trade paperback | ISBN 9798889844075 ebook
Subjects: LCSH: Body image | Body weight—Social aspects | Thin people | Eating disorders—Prevention | Self-acceptance
Classification: LCC BF697.5.B63 L43 2026 (print) | LCC BF697.5.B63 (ebook)
LC record available at https://lccn.loc.gov/2026001313
LC ebook record available at https://lccn.loc.gov/2026001314

1 2 3 4 5 6 7 8 9 MARQUIS 30 29 28 27 26

Printed in Canada

To my parents

and

To my sister, Manue

The body is not a thing, it is a situation—it is our grasp on the world and the sketch of our projects.

—SIMONE DE BEAUVOIR, *The Second Sex*

Contents

Introduction

Spinning. The bathroom is spinning around me as I sit crouched on the floor. Swirls of white and silver. I clutch the edge of the toilet bowl to vomit.

I am drunk.

It's a Monday night. I haven't gone partying. That's not the reason.

I am drunk and vomiting in my bathroom because I have had two sangrias and only two tiny falafel balls for dinner. I have been restricting food.

Ten minutes later, I get up from the floor and walk on shaky limbs to my bedroom. It's 9 p.m. I'm supposed to take my dog, Carol, out for her final walk of the night.

I am so sick that I can't get out of bed for another hour. I toss and turn to keep myself awake until the spinning stops, until I feel steady enough to leash her, take the elevator down to the first floor, and guide her to the tree a couple of steps from the front door. There she pees, and then we go back up to the apartment. This is a five-minute routine, yet I couldn't do it in my drunkenness.

Buildings collapse. Bridges collapse. People collapse. And so do worlds. When they do, we lose our bearings. Either we die in defeat or find a new way to live. As I crawl back into bed and collapse, and Carol curls into a ball in the crook of my knees, I know I've lost my bearings.

I have failed Carol. This is my first time failing her as her caretaker. If I love her, then I must change. I must return to eating disorder counseling. I don't care about myself. Not at this moment. Returning has nothing to do with caring for myself. This is for Carol.

THIS STORY, or some version of it, might be familiar to you. Perhaps you have dieted to the point of developing a full-fledged eating disorder. Or perhaps you've struggled to lose weight and been discouraged because you never could achieve the slender silhouettes of the models or movie stars you admire. Perhaps you've watched someone you love struggle to fit into a shape that was not theirs. Regardless of the particulars, you've experienced the damage of our longstanding fixation on thinness.

This obsession isn't new. In the past thirty years alone, we've seen the "heroin chic" vogue of the 1990s migrate to the online "thinspo" blogs of the 2000s and 2010s, and now, in the 2020s, these blogs have morphed into the communities following #SkinnyTok and its sisters on social media. As someone who has lived through these shifts, I know firsthand how badly the thinness ideal can harm us. And as someone who has tried to grapple with it as a philosopher, I've long wondered how we can overthrow "the tyranny of slenderness"—an expression coined by feminist thinker Kim Chernin.[1] At the heart of this book lies a difficult question: *How can we resist this tyranny, given its seemingly unending return?*

My answer draws on my experience struggling with and ultimately recovering from eating issues and on the most current accounts of "diet culture" and its relationship to eating disorders. Each of this book's chapters begins and ends with a vignette from my life, and in between explores theories of cultural critics and social philosophers of interest to anyone combating the thinness ideal. If you're curious about combating this punishing beauty standard and want to envision a world where we relate to our bodies in empowering ways, then you will find valuable ideas in this book.

In its simplest form, my thesis is this: Changing your physique—whether through diet, exercise, cosmetics, or surgeries—to conform with beauty standards will *never* bring you true pleasure or lasting happiness, despite the false claims by diet culture and the beauty industry. Only alternative ways of thinking about your body, combined with your own suite of practices for *being in* your body, will deliver the pleasure and happiness you deserve.

In developing this argument, I make and explore three supporting claims. The first is that promoting more inclusive beauty standards is one important step, but not enough on its own to combat the body dissatisfaction that leads us to obsessively focus on how we look to others. Our bodies are more than objects that are sized up according to external standards. So—and this is my second, complementary claim—instead of merely widening what counts as a beautiful body *as an object* when viewed by others, we need a whole new way to listen to and care for our bodies from the inside out, *as subjects*. If we do not find this new way, then the tyranny of thinness, and other oppressive ways to distract us from the self-care we need to flourish, will keep coming back again and again. My third claim is that this new way of thinking and being is not achieved in isolation: Dismantling oppression is always more effectively done as part of a community, connected with and actively exploring the ways other people achieve their own success stories with self-care. For this third claim, I "show by doing": I invite you to join me in celebrating several communities of resistance—writers, activists, bodyworkers, artists, and those from so many other walks of life—that offer you a plurality of ways to achieve self-care.

By the end of this book, you will have tools to cultivate greater body acceptance, despite the ongoing onslaught of messages meant to inspire us to shrink ourselves. In addition, while thinness has stuck stubbornly as a norm for decades, my reasoning applies to combating other punitive beauty standards that you and people you love may be dealing with.

Why should we take time to study and evaluate the slenderness ideal today? If you were reading these lines in the 2010s, you might have considered embracing body positivity, an ethos championing self-love and diversity in beauty, as a remedy to your struggles with the slenderness ideal. Then body-positive activists promoted overcoming the shame we experience from not living up to our stringent beauty standards—standards that typically elevated a young, slim physique, without visible disabilities, as the norm. Yet the movement came under attack: Did fashion companies capitalize on consumer interest in diversity just to sell more clothes and cosmetics? Did they really care about being inclusive? And who can summon a sunny attitude about their physique now that trends like #legginglegs or "yacht shoulders" are blanketing our social media feeds? So enthusiasm for the body positivity movement has ebbed. But I have a way to take its core idea of self-love and bring it back in a form that can last.

In the 2020s, the cosmetic use of GLP-1 medications, such as Ozempic and Wegovy, has further enshrined the thinness ideal and sparked debates about the "death of body positivity." Yet if we pull back, we see that drugs for weight loss have long existed: amphetamines in the 1950s and fen-phen in the 1990s. People have also turned to cigarettes and even ADHD medication to curb their appetite. This wider angle can help us identify earlier versions of the turn to appetite suppressants and stimulants, and to anticipate future ones. Of course, GLP-1s are lifesaving for many: They've become game-changers for people who have medical conditions, such as diabetes, or whose weight issues are taking a significant toll on their health. As someone who has wrestled with the thinness ideal for decades, however, I worry about using these medications for reasons purely motivated by this ideal. You might find yourself in the same position, or you may be the parent or teacher of someone coming of age in these conditions. Should we do everything possible to become slim—whether by dieting or using medications that come with a long list of side effects? If not, what other options do we have?

Before laying out a strategy to address these questions, let me say a few words about why I can help you reflect on them. First, as someone who has written on toxic beauty standards for over a decade and has recovered from restrictive eating, I know how damaging body image issues can be and how freeing it can be to overcome them. In my case, I occupied a middle ground that Jennifer Thomas and Jenni Schaefer call "almost anorexic" in their book by the same name.[2] Because I was never extremely ill nor lost an excessive amount of weight, it was hard for me to recognize I had a problem with eating and to seek treatment. Not only that, but it was difficult to see myself as a survivor for the purposes of writing this book. I've hesitated to claim the authority necessary for writing *personally* about disordered eating. Nevertheless, I now recognize that my preoccupation with my body size and eating habits exceeded what is common. I almost wrote "normal" instead of "common." If I had, I might have given the impression that our collective body dissatisfaction and the diet culture that preys on it are natural and unavoidable. They aren't.

Second, thanks to my training in philosophy, I can speak to a broader set of concerns than those narrated in eating disorder recovery memoirs or discussed in empirical studies. Memoirs of this kind usually focus on the specific triggers that set off a pattern of disordered eating and the journey the author took to overcome their disorder. Empirical research provides data, including the prevalence of body dissatisfaction in a population or the correlation between this dissatisfaction and dieting. Additionally, such research can teach us about the successes of different strategies, such as media literacy, to overcome negative body image.

Philosophy can draw on this data, but it offers something different. Philosophy has something to say about *what a body is.* The powerful ideas I draw on in philosophy teach us that the body is not merely a hunk of matter. It's the origin of our intentional movements, the vantage point through which we perceive the world, and an entity embedded in the chains of causes and effects that define life itself. In addition, the body is an object in the eyes of others. But by focusing on how we appear to those around us, we forget that our bodies are subjects: teaching us when we need food, when we're ill, and when we need a sense of security.

The chapters of *The Tyranny of Thinness* fall into two parts. The first is an analysis of the thinness ideal, while the second part consists of recommendations to better safeguard us against it. When faced with any type of problem, the first thing to do is to stop and analyze what is going on. Whether it's a look behind your washing machine to see why it's rattling or an X-ray to determine whether your ankle is broken, we take an "analytical" approach to our concerns every day. Likewise, in the first part of this book, we'll put on our philosophical lenses, so to speak, to understand where the thinness aesthetic came from and why it has come back so many times. Specifically, we'll consider how children absorb beauty ideals; how girls and people who were socialized as girls, in particular, begin to objectify themselves at puberty; how diet culture and beauty culture can harm us; how the thinness ideal has evolved in recent decades; how the body positivity movement offered hope in the face of the slenderness ideal; and how the COVID-19 pandemic intensified disordered eating. Although not all women will identify with the experience of "girlhood" depicted here, the burdens of diet culture and the beauty industry are ones that many of us face.

Once we have a good look at the problem, we can then turn to solutions to it. That's why part 2 canvasses ways to resist the tyranny of thinness. We'll delve into the promise of self-care and intuitive eating; mindful movement; the power of physical pleasure; and remaking the world to resist diet culture. The solutions we'll probe in this part stem from my personal experience, other narratives about reconnecting with food and our bodies, and psychological research.

Throughout this book, I'll share my story to inspire you to craft your own. The idea that helped me recover was the notion of self-care. Ancient philosophy prized caring for the self in many forms. Whether it was about sexuality, nutrition, physical exercise, meditation, or intellectual activity, philosophy has had a long and often underappreciated history of reflecting on self-care. I want to reconnect with this tradition of philosophical thinking, but with a twist. "Care of the self" in Antiquity was primarily reserved for male elites. Here, I'll reveal how important self-care is not only for women who have suffered from disordered eating or negative body image, but also for each one of us—regardless of our body size, our gender, our sexuality, our race, our age, or our physical abilities. In her writings on wrestling with cancer, the feminist thinker Audre Lorde famously proclaimed self-care to be an "act of political warfare."[3] For her, embracing self-care challenged the notion that lives like hers were expendable. Like Lorde, I want my experience as a queer woman of color to speak to the value of caring for oneself.

The stakes are high: Body dissatisfaction predicts disordered eating and other mental health conditions. That's why it's more urgent than ever to fight back. Let's reject comparing our bodies to those of others, and let's teach younger generations to do the same. Let's practice intuitive eating and other forms of self-care. Let's endorse flexible beauty ideals. And let's create spaces that accommodate a wide range of body types, including those with physical disabilities. Let's work to create the conditions to thrive in our bodies.

The Tyranny of Thinness bridges the philosophical and the practical, the personal and the political, the individual and the social. Each of our bodies bears a history within it, and each of our bodies has a story to tell. My book is an invitation for you to write *and* rewrite your own story.

PART 1

Thin Is In (Yet) Again

1

Lessons Learned and Unlearned

Taught from their infancy that beauty is woman's sceptre, the mind shapes itself to the body, and, roaming round its gilt cage, only seeks to adorn its prison.

—MARY WOLLSTONECRAFT, *A Vindication of the Rights of Women*

Though her hands are gnarled from arthritis, my grandmother kneads the dough with quick and vigorous squeezes, and teaches me to do the same. Mamie Maude, as I call her, is showing me how to make tarte aux myrtilles (blueberry tart). The only way for me to reach the bowl is to stand on a stool that occupies the end of my parents' narrow Manhattan kitchen. Once the dough has been kneaded, I climb down from the stool. We let the dough rest as we struggle to pick the remaining sticky pieces from our fingers.

A few hours later, we remove the dough from the bowl. Then comes the fun of stretching it, laying it out on a pie pan, and then pinching the edges to form creases. The game is challenging, but I then get my reward: Mamie lets me add in the berries. I grab them in handfuls from the container and let them crash in blue cascades onto the crust. I love that part more than anything.

At dinner, I eat my slice with joy—and no table manners. I love the tarts we cook together, as well as the beignets and the crêpes we make on summer afternoons. Photos of me with blueberry smothered around my face all the way up my cheeks fill my childhood family albums. Alongside several pictures of me with ice cream dripping down my face.

Mamie dies in 1995. I am nine years old.

THE DAYS I enjoyed baking with Mamie would be my last moments of innocence. With her, food was a source of pleasure, and cooking well was an accomplishment. The familial and societal messages about eating that I would later absorb destroyed these early lessons. I learned that eating is dangerous because it leads to the worst of all sins—being fat—and that food restriction is the only way to avoid this danger. My experience raises a question that is relevant for many of us: *Why do we lose our "native" eating habits?*

This question will guide us in this chapter. As I mentioned in the preface, we must first don our philosophical lenses to analyze how the thinness ideal affects us, before sketching solutions that resist it. We'll study the connection between this ideal and dieting and then ask *why* thinness emerged as a beauty standard for girls and women. Along the way, we'll touch on psychological accounts of body image and disordered eating, as well as philosophical "genealogies"—or what you might simply call "histories"—of the slenderness ideal.

Hate Your Body? Then Diet!

The fact that I developed image issues at the age of about nine is unsurprising: Psychologists have concluded that girls as young as five show preferences for "thinner ideal body sizes than their perceived current size."[1] As a girl, I also began to fear body fat. Perhaps you did, too, if you are a reader who resonates with the change I am characterizing—from food as a joy without restriction to food as dangerous and requiring control. Children often begin to idealize thinness by listening to what teens and adults say about their own bodies and others, and grow "sensitive to cultural pressures to conform to a limited range of acceptable body shapes."[2] Remarks from relatives, bullying on the schoolyard, or worshipping models or actors can lure us into hating our body.

This hatred has a more innocuous name: *negative body image.* The term "body image" itself refers to many phenomena: size and weight perception, size and weight satisfaction, appearance satisfaction, investment in appearance, body acceptance, and others. To simplify, I have in mind what body image expert Sarah Grogan defines as "a person's perceptions, thoughts, and feelings about his or her body."[3] For example, researchers may study the prevalence of anabolic steroid use and people's appearance-focused motivations for using this type of drug. Or psychologists may analyze the influence of our media consumption and media literacy on our feelings about our body.

So a negative body image, or body dissatisfaction, usually stems from a "perceived discrepancy between a person's evaluation of his or her body and his or her ideal body," according to Grogan.[4] For instance, when test subjects view images of the human body and are asked to choose the one matching their current body type, and the one closest to their ideal one, women reliably choose a figure slimmer than their own. This difference shows that they are dissatisfied with their body type. And in questionnaire and interview studies, girls and women often report being unhappy with the size of their breasts or the levels of fat in their legs, abdomen, and buttocks.[5]

Like many girls and women, I became unhappy with my body by idealizing the waifish models and actresses of my generation. Even at my lowest adult weight, I never felt at peace with my body. How could I? Didn't every morsel of food I consumed threaten my efforts to stay slender? In my mid-teens, I came across the Duchess of Windsor's quip "You can never be too rich or too thin" in a book on women's health. Though the book criticized her statement, I was left unmoved. Instead of seeing the danger in her one-liner, I grew obsessed with my body's size. Year by year, the thinness ideal, however closely I embodied it, preyed on me. For instance, in my early thirties, I gained and lost the same 5 pounds again and again to keep myself at my "ideal weight": between 125 and 130 pounds. I am six feet tall, so that meant being in the "underweight" BMI category.

BMI, or body mass index, has many imperfections as a metric. It's based on a person's height and weight and does not consider their proportion of fat vs. muscle, where the fat is distributed on their body, or their metabolic health. It was developed nearly two centuries ago by the mathematician Aldophe Quetelet, who sought to understand the characteristics of the "normal man." He did not intend these statistics as a tool for diagnosing health conditions. Moreover, his averages were based on the measurements of white men and might have little relevance to other racial groups.[6] That said, these criticisms have primarily targeted the issue of classifying people as "overweight" or "obese." On the other end of the spectrum, the World Health Organization also has worries about BMI: "The cut-off point of 18.5 for underweight in both genders has less experimental validity as a cut-off point for moderate and severe thinness but is a reasonable value for use pending further, comprehensive studies."[7] In my experience, once I lost enough weight to count as moderately thin, as I did when I felt faint after two drinks, I knew that I had reached a level of thinness that jeopardized my health. Despite the BMI's flaws, and whether or not we're defined as underweight, the weight-cycling that prevails these days reveals how much we struggle with our bodies.

To keep our weight "in check," many of us turn to dieting. Although this behavior may mean different things to different people, it generally includes "an intentional, often temporary, change in eating to achieve weight loss."[8] Psychologists have observed that there's a strong correlation between body dissatisfaction and "weight control practices."[9] One study showed that female adolescents were at high risk for feeling body dissatisfaction and using unhealthy weight control practices, "most likely because of strong societal pressures emphasizing thinness."[10] But dieting can occur before adolescence. Girls as young as six try to control their body size by restricting food.

"Body dissatisfaction has been reported in 50% of children aged 6–12 years," one recent study reported. "Girls and boys have also been shown to be significantly invested in thin and muscular ideals by 5–9 years old, while 29% of girls aged 10–14 years have reported attempting to lose weight."[11]

The association between body dissatisfaction and dieting as a solution to this dissatisfaction is worrisome. Researchers in psychology have noted that the biggest contributing risk factors for developing disordered eating behaviors include body dissatisfaction and extreme weight control behaviors.[12] Philosophers have made similar claims. For example, in her article "Sublime Hunger: A Consideration of Eating Disorders Beyond Beauty," Sheila Lintott writes that many girls and women begin to diet to conform to the norm of feminine thinness, but for some, this dieting morphs into anorexia or bulimia. Our efforts to be slim can become attempts to curb our appetite for its own sake, Lintott says. Eventually, appearance concerns ebb and give way to a fixation on controlling food intake and hunger (more on this in chapter 6).

It's worth emphasizing the other culprits in the development of eating disorders—genetic tendencies, psychological traits such as perfectionism, and higher depressiveness can also predict anorexia.[13] Eating-disorder memoirs, such as Marya Hornbacher's critically acclaimed *Wasted*, highlight the complex genesis of disordered eating behaviors. After her move to Minnesota at the age of eight, in an environment where her parents often fought, Hornbacher started engaging in bulimic behavior. As the stresses of adolescence, intertwined with her ambitions as a writer, took hold, her bulimia then gave way to anorexia. During her schooling at the elite Interlochen Center for the Arts, she found herself surrounded by equally ambitious young women who engaged in extreme dieting. Food restriction no longer felt like a means to mold her appearance, but more of a "habit" she couldn't shake. She repeatedly starved herself out of a deeply rooted desire for self-destruction. Her narrative shows how family history, educational settings, and individual psychological characteristics coalesce. Yet

Hornbacher herself believes that the "cultural environment is an equal, if not greater, culprit in the *popularity* of eating disorders."[14] For her, eating disorders are an expression of self-destructiveness in a society that elevates thinness as a "strange state of grace."[15] Her memoir does not point to a single incident that led to her battle with her body and food. In some cases, however, acute childhood trauma can also trigger problematic eating habits, more often binging than anorexia.[16] For example, Roxane Gay, in her memoir *Hunger*, writes that being sexually assaulted at a young age precipitated years of binge-eating for her.

But please note that disordered eating affects people across the board, regardless of gender, race, sexuality, or age. Although we may still call to mind a white teenage girl when we think of anorexia or bulimia, we're inadvertently reinforcing a stereotype. We might assume that certain populations are not affected by eating disorders, but this is mistaken. Increasing attention is being paid to restrictive eating in boys and men. Although girls and women are still more likely to develop anorexia or bulimia, the rate of these eating disorders among males is now rising more quickly than among their female counterparts.[17] Likewise, people of color are just as likely to experience disordered eating as white people—but are about half as likely to have it diagnosed.[18]

LGBTQ+ individuals also wrestle with disordered eating. Gay and bisexual boys do so at rates four times higher than heterosexual peers, and lesbian and bisexual girls twice as high, according to the National Association of Anorexia Nervosa and Associated Disorders. The association's report also draws attention to the fact that "32% of transgender people report using their eating disorder to modify their body without hormones, such as to reduce curves or halt menstruation."[19] The struggles of middle-aged and older persons are also gaining more attention: Going through life transitions such as menopause and children leaving home can intensify people's disordered eating.[20] Research has also documented these shifts and the difficulties older persons face in receiving eating disorder treatment. A 2017 study conducted in the UK found that "evidence that lifetime and active EDs [eating disorders] are common amongst women in mid-life, compounded by the lack of healthcare access and treatment."[21] My experience speaks to these facts. I'm a queer Black woman, and I suffered at my worst in my thirties. So let's ditch our assumptions and stock images of disordered eating.

In my case, I can't pinpoint a singular event—such as a divorce in my family, a crush's rejection, or bullying—that pushed me to undereat. Rather, each magazine article after the other and, later, each thinspo ("thinspiration," or admiration of excessively thin bodies) blog post after the other would drain all joy I had around cooking and eating. For me, the pressure I felt to consider a career in modeling further tipped the scales. My mother first implanted the idea after having professional photographs taken of my sister and me. Later, acquaintances and even strangers told me that I should model. As I'll describe in chapter 3, I was flattered and pursued the possibility in my late teens. I could not anticipate, of course, that this pressure would eventually lead me to an eating disorder.

Chasing thinness may be the most ubiquitous way we pursue beauty today. Our efforts to "look good" often stem from wanting to "fit in." And we try to fit in by measuring ourselves against others. Philosophers have long acknowledged the harms of social comparisons. In the eighteenth century, the French thinker Jean-Jacques Rousseau thought that we're born good but society has a corrupting influence that pushes us to compare ourselves to others. He distinguished between "amour propre" (self-esteem) and "amour de soi" (self-love). Amour propre is a form of self-esteem grounded in the opinions of others: We stake our self-worth on what people around us say. We become "too ugly" only by filtering our body through the gaze of others. These days, especially for women, that usually means "too fat," but in different times and cultures, it could mean not living up to other norms. Amour de soi, on the other hand, motivates us to care for our well-being: basic needs, such as food and shelter. We love ourselves because we have an instinctive desire to thrive.

Today researchers in psychology use different terms than Rousseau did: A "tripartite influence model" of three factors—friends, family, and media—affect how we view our body (more on this in chapter 2). But the heart of Rousseau's observation remains the same. Whether we're talking about slimness or some other beauty norm, we need to learn to loosen the hold of social comparisons and embrace the power of caring for ourselves. This may be easier said than done, but I'll narrate a path toward such self-care in part 2 of this book.

Why Do We Care About Thinness?

To better understand how the thinness ideal burdens us, we need to tackle an important question: Why do we care so much about being thin? After all, you might have seen early representations of plump fertility goddesses or Peter Paul Rubens's portraits of robust women. What happened?

One interesting line of thinking involves the idea of "distinction," a concept that can help us see how thinness as an ideal has evolved in specific eras and cultures. Twentieth-century French philosopher Pierre Bourdieu originated the notion of distinction: "Social subjects . . . distinguish themselves by the distinctions they make, between the beautiful and the ugly, the distinguished and the vulgar, in which their position in the objective classifications is expressed or betrayed."[22] That's quite the mouthful! In simpler terms, we try to cement our place in society by developing features that mark us as better than others. Leanness is one such characteristic. And in our society, people seek to "distinguish themselves by cultivating tastes, diets, and physical appearances that are in opposition to those of the subordinated groups," writes sociologist Sabrina Strings in her book *Fearing the Black Body: The Racial Origins of Fatphobia.*[23] She explains that fatphobia is rooted in racism.

Strings notes that in the Renaissance era, Europeans favored symmetry, proportion, and a certain amount of fat in bodies both white and Black. But with the seventeenth century came a new figure: the "thin, fine" European man. He distinguished himself from those who were inferior and beholden to their appetites—that is, people of African descent, whom he defined as gluttons. Consider Rubens, whose paintings of women gave rise to our popular term "Rubenesque." Rubens himself was a thin man who, according to Strings, "lamented the fatness of so-called modern men."[24] Likewise, René Descartes, the French philosopher famed for his statement "I think; therefore, I am," was known to eat little and to advise against overindulgence. And across the English Channel, doctors began to complain about expanding waistlines, sustained by the introduction of sugar into European diets.

The thinness ideal then extended to white women in the eighteenth century and became an emblem of middle- and upper-class femininity. The rise of female slenderness in Europe paralleled efforts to stereotype African women. Take the notorious example of Saartjie "Sara" Baartman, who was displayed in exhibitions across Europe starting in 1806. Known as "the Hottentot Venus," Baartman was "promoted as an erotic and scientific curiosity."[25] Visitors could view her and, for an additional fee, could touch her body. By claiming she was the archetype of beauty among the Hottentots, all the while mocking her body, these exhibitions helped cast Black bodies as ugly and Black beauty norms as primitive.

The United States adopted these European associations. White Americans connected Blackness with gross appetites and fatness. Periodicals, such as *Godey's Lady's Book* and *Harper's Bazaar*, called on (white) women to be slender. Criticisms of the influx of migrants from Southern and Eastern Europe helped reinforce the whiteness/leanness equation: Americans classified new migrants as non-white and criticized them for their physiques and supposed gluttony. Although doctors sometimes worried about the effects of excessive slimness on fertility during this period, fatphobia still took hold of the American imagination.

Currently, glamour seems synonymous with thinness in girls and women. That's the link I internalized growing up in the '90s. But how did we get there? Let's pick up where Strings's history leaves off and turn to the US in the twentieth century.

From the 1940s onward, the fashion industry intensified the link between thinness and beauty. As sociologist and writer Elizabeth Wissinger describes in *This Year's Model,* the standardization of clothing sizes laid the ground for the standardization of the measurements of fashion models, such as weight and height requirements. "The new corporeality demanded by industrialized perception pulled for serially interchangeable models, with identical proportions portraying this attenuated ideal. Those who did not fit the standard were eventually winnowed out," Wissinger writes. Designers preferred featuring one body type in their shows and advertising. The prevailing view that taller and thinner models best showcased clothing motivated designers to elevate lean bodies. John Robert Powers, one of the leaders in championing the idea of a "professional model," said: "The tall, slight figure complements the lines of clothes and makes them more effective . . . A short girl has a stubby effect in photography and cannot display clothes to the best advantage . . . In other words, they must be tall and slim, well-proportioned and able to handle their bodies with perfect control and a maximum of grace."[26]

In Western societies, the obviously one-sided point of view that Powers held still holds sway over how we think of beautiful bodies. Today we continue to worship thinness, and discrimination against fat persons, often under the pretext of health concerns, runs rampant.* We equate fatness with being unhealthy and disparage those who are fat. As Kate Manne describes in her 2024 book *Unshrinking: How to Face Fatphobia,* there may be correlations between high body fat and certain illnesses, but these correlations don't imply causation.[27] Manne cites a range of studies that challenge the link between fatness and unhealthiness, such as one that found being physically active mattered more than having a so-called normal BMI for reducing the risk of cardiovascular disease.[28] Manne concludes that people mistake fatness as the biggest problem when, in fact, physical fitness and other factors matter as much to our health. While I

* I want to note that in referring to "fat persons" or "fatness" in this book, I'm using these expressions as value-neutral descriptions of people and their body types.

do not mean to underestimate the evidence that being overweight can lead to metabolic dysfunction and other health problems, the research makes us pause to question our often reflexive associations between body size, weight, and health. Manne adds that some fat persons will avoid the doctor when they need treatment because they fear being lectured about their weight, thus delaying any medical interventions. Or on the flip side, if they do seek care, they'll find their concerns overlooked while doctors zero in on their fatness. Many people also live with the shame that stems from our moralization of fatness. Rather than being a neutral descriptor of someone's body type, fatness signifies lesser worth in society and gets shamed. Such body shame, to borrow from the work of philosopher Luna Dolezal, can become *limiting.*[29] That is, it threatens those who suffer from it from leading flourishing lives.

You might think of body shame as a problem for girls and women in the US and Europe. Unfortunately, alongside other exports, the West's slenderness obsession has spread across the globe. For example, before glamorous representations of thin bodies reached certain cultures, anorexia and bulimia were almost nonexistent. A noteworthy example is the introduction of Western TV shows to Fiji in the 1990s. "In 1995, without television, girls in Fiji appeared to be free of the eating disorders common in the West. But by 1998, after just a few years of sexy soap operas and seductive commercials, 11.3 percent of adolescent girls reported they at least once had purged to lose weight. Disorders increased in girls and women in Fiji," as per the pioneering work of Harvard Medical School psychiatrist Anne E. Becker.[30] Although some researchers are cautious in claiming that eating disorders are culture-bound, both psychological studies and anthropological evidence give reason to think that Western aesthetic norms have influenced the rise of eating disorders outside the West.

Today, around the world, women feel the pressure to be slim, while more men want to develop a toned and muscular physique.[31] Both standards encourage us to have a lean body type, with different emphases for each gender. These ideals continue to shift, with a heightened expectation today that women should also appear toned. Boys and men are increasingly suffering the effects of dieting and struggling with disordered eating, so why are girls and women still more likely to engage in weight-loss dieting and more prone to anorexia and bulimia? To better grapple with the specific problem of glorifying female slenderness, let's have a look at the feminist thinkers Naomi Wolf and Susan Bordo.

The Thinness Ideal: A Reaction to Women's Progress?

In her 1990 book *The Beauty Myth*, Naomi Wolf describes how beauty culture, including diet culture, can be seen as a backlash to the second wave of feminism. In this period from the 1960s to the early 1980s, feminists advocated equality in employment, politics, marriage, family, education, and sexuality. Their activism in the United States led to achievements like the Equal Pay Act of 1963, Title IX in 1972, and the legalization of abortion through the US Supreme Court's ruling on *Roe v. Wade* in 1973 (later overturned in 2022). After this wave of feminism passed, beauty became a "political weapon" wielded to stop women's advancement and served as a "counterforce . . . operating to checkmate the inheritance of feminism on every level in the lives of Western women," Wolf says.[32] Despite the rights they won in the 1960s and '70s, women faced new burdens with the costly diets, cosmetic products, and surgeries necessary to comply with beauty standards. The imposing demands of having flawless skin, impeccable hair, manicured nails, stylish clothes, and a slim body replaced the overturned legal restrictions. While men could climb the corporate ladder with little attention to their appearance, women needed to be both successful *and* attractive. Instead of the traditional double shift of paid and domestic labor, women incurred a "third shift": beauty work.

Consider the disproportionate use of aesthetic surgeries by women as compared to men. When Wolf was writing in 1990, procedures such as "tummy tucks" and breast augmentations were soaring in popularity, and procedures on men were far less common. And despite earning less overall than men, women allotted more of their income to buying cosmetics, purchasing gym memberships, attending Weight Watchers programs, and, for some, going under the knife. To be clear, Wolf doesn't shun the idea of celebrating human beauty. She worries, however, about the extreme measures that many women take to comply with beauty standards. The dieting that goes hand in hand with the obsession with feminine slenderness is one such measure: Hunger trails women in the throes of this obsession, with binges, guilt, and endless weight cycling, close on its heels.

In *Unbearable Weight*, published three years later, Susan Bordo views anorexia and everyday preoccupations with being slim as continuous with one another. She attributes gender associations between women and slenderness to several factors. After the feminist liberation movements of the 1960s and '70s, girls and young women started expressing fear of and dislike for society's traditional roles for women.[33] They didn't want to be like their mothers, working in lesser jobs or catering to the interests of men. Alongside emerged "a deep fear of 'the Female,' with all its more nightmarish and archetypal association of voracious hunger and sexual insatiability."[34] Recall the historical tropes about women as "praying mantises" ready to suck a man of his vitality. Newly emancipated women wanted to separate themselves from these associations. They found themselves torn between two contradictory images: Although they saw themselves as productive and capable of mastery, they also fought the stereotype of femininity as consumption. Bordo describes some anorexic adolescents' disgust of the female body: They feel disdain for "womanly" bodies. Some go so far as to express the wish to remain children forever. Dieting becomes the necessary step to take to achieve a waifish figure. This leads to a paradox: Our culture praises women for their power over their bodies and appetites, all the while selling a form of self-control that ultimately disempowers them. As I learned, painfully, the night I couldn't care for my dog, there's only so long we can survive on two falafel balls for dinner.

Altogether, the theories we've just explored show how praising restrained eating and demonizing body fat sowed our focus on thinness. While we have seen increasing body diversity in fashion and media since the 2010s, the tyranny of thinness still dominates. High-end runway fashion in the 2020s continues to showcase very skinny models.[35] And this trend now runs even stronger thanks to the cosmetic uses of GLP-1s.

Can We Change Our Beauty Standards? Or Are We Stuck with Thinness?

I've described the evolution of our norms about body fat to illustrate what a genealogy of beauty standards looks like. We could make similar arguments about other norms: fetishizing pale skin in the first part of the twentieth century, expectations about body hair in various societies, or the elevation of physical markers of Caucasian heritage in the West, like straight hair.

The first lesson from these genealogies is that standards of beauty have evolved across human history, and vary across the globe. Not everything about our aesthetic norms is fixed by our nature. Even if today's norms about body size and fatness seem entrenched, they've had variations across time and place. Philosophers call such norms *socially constructed.* That is, natural features don't (fully) determine their content; instead, cultural influences shape them. For example, thinness has been equated with sickliness, poverty, and ugliness in societies where food is scarce. There, a certain amount of body fat becomes a sign of health and wealth, as well as beauty. Scientists are quick to point out that certain features do seem to be universally valued, such as clear skin and symmetrical facial features. Our preference for these features likely has evolutionary origins, as clear skin and symmetry have been theorized to be connected to fertility.[36] Yet in the case of body fat, the standards are more malleable and tied to cultural factors. At times, women's body fat has been understood as a sign of a good partner to procreate with. Those who subscribe to an evolutionary view of beauty point out that a curved waist has long signaled reproductive fitness.[37]

The second lesson from these genealogies is simple, too. Because beauty standards are flexible, we can change them! We can resist oppressive aesthetic norms, such as the overbearing pressure to be slim, and we can create new standards. We can also challenge the idea that beauty should play as important a role in our lives as it does today.

That said, the bar for challenging the thinness ideal is getting higher. In *Perfect Me: Beauty as an Ethical Ideal*, the philosopher Heather Widdows explains that this ideal is becoming increasingly prevalent, and while it can take different forms across the globe, it remains one of the primary standards women feel the need to live up to. From being catwalk-thin to slim with curves, or athletic and buff, "slimness in some form is crucial," she writes.[38] I have seen this play out since my teenage years across the places where I've lived. In New York City and Paris in the 1990s and 2000s, the standard was skinny. Yet as I write these words in Miami in 2025, the norm is slimness with curves and a certain amount of muscle tone. Widdows also claims that beauty has become such a dominant ideal that women derive much of their self-worth from their appearance and invest a lot of time and money in perfecting it (more on this in chapter 3). Her work raises an important concern about our predicament: Since the slimness norm now has such a tight grip on us cross-culturally, can we even shake it anymore?

I'm optimistic that we can meet this challenge. Yet this will take more than simply telling girls and women that "every body is beautiful" or encouraging them to declare "I love my body" every morning as they step out of the shower. We can only achieve long-lasting change if we offer a viable alternative to toxic beauty standards. What we need, and what I hope my journey will show, is that embracing self-care can help us move beyond the pressure to be slender and find a better ideal. Instead of valuing our body only for its appearance, we can also learn to appreciate it for its functionality and the pleasure it affords, as I'll explain in part 2. But before getting there, let's use my own experience as an example of how diet and beauty culture take hold of teenage girls and women.

I've just turned thirteen and entered a lycée (secondary school) in Paris. With this change comes the freedom to eat what I want at lunchtime. There is no cafeteria at my high school; my classmates and I either bring food from home or roam the streets off the Champs-Élysées in search of a meal. I opt for a pain au chocolat. Over the past year, I've begun hearing that I should model. I've also seen how skinny the girls on the runway are, and I've heard of their tiny meals. To look like them, I'll need to eat less. Much less than the sandwiches and desserts I enjoyed when my mother made lunch for me. I'm still growing and want to be as tall as possible. I must eat something. The compromise: pain au chocolat, my favorite breakfast food. Sure, it isn't a plain yogurt or piece of fruit. In the shiny magazines I devour every month, I've learned that models live off these foods. But a pain au chocolat is enough to get through afternoon lessons and allow my growth spurt. Right?

I peel off the bread crust and nibble on it, little by little, until I reach the best part: the chocolate center. I take quick bites, savoring the blend of sweetness and the twinge of bitterness from the dark cocoa, all the while hoping the taste will linger into the afternoon. I'm still hungry, but I open a book and wait at the patisserie until it's time to return to class.

As someone who came of age in the late 1990s and early 2000s, I equated beauty with slenderness and dieting. And if you're of the same generation, I bet you did, too. These associations made us believe that we needed to be thin, and today they're continuing to affect young girls and teens. Adolescence is a period that heightens the body dissatisfaction many girls already have. As their body evolves, the weight they put on often makes them further depart from ultra-thin beauty standards. This combination lays the groundwork for a precipitous increase in eating disorders. As is well-documented, the prevalence of these conditions skyrockets between the ages of twelve and fifteen.[39] In my case, these years would undo everything wholesome I had embodied about eating and cooking. Shame would replace all the pride I had in preparing meals, and fear would replace all the pleasure food afforded. And amid this, my unhappiness with my weight would grow unchecked. That's when I unlearned the lessons that I had learned from Mamie.

2

Girlhood, or the Shock of Seeing Yourself Seen

"At thirteen, I walked around bare-legged, in a short dress," another woman told me. "A man, sniggering, made a comment about my fat calves. The next day, my mother made me wear stockings and lengthen my skirt, but I will never forget the shock I suddenly felt in seeing myself seen." The little girl feels as though her body is escaping her, that it is no longer the clear expression of her individuality; it becomes foreign to her; and at the same moment, she is grasped by others as a thing; in the street, eyes follow her; her body is subject to comments; she would like to become invisible; she is afraid of her flesh and afraid to show her flesh.

—SIMONE DE BEAUVOIR, *The Second Sex*

I'm twelve or thirteen when I buy a coral crop top from Petit Bateau, a French clothing store for children and teens. I don't remember why my mother let me have one. All I remember about the shirt is that one day, when I'm sitting hunched at a desk, my stomach folds over. My father looks at me. Does he see the same folds that I see?

That split-second moment still lives in my memory twenty-five years later. If there is any place on my body I obsess about, it's my waist.

But two years into living in Miami, I succumb to the local fad of wearing crop tops and acquire my first one since my teenage years. The first time I walk out into the street wearing it, I feel naked. No one seems to pay attention to my body: neither do I notice anyone's gaze, nor do I get catcalled. Still, I can't shake the impression that I've stepped out of my home without a vital item of clothing, as though I were roaming Miami without underwear and pants on. The feeling of exposure fades, though. My vanity gets the better of me, and I think I look cute in it. I purchase two more within a few months, and then two others a year later.

Whenever I bend over when wearing a crop top, I never forget to suck my stomach in. My flesh can't fold over. The shame of that moment is indelible.

AT PUBERTY, many girls and people socialized as girls find themselves the target of unwanted scrutiny. I did, and you might have, too. For the first time, we experience the "shock" of seeing ourselves *seen*, as described by Simone de Beauvoir in the passage that opens this chapter. In *The Second Sex*, her landmark feminist book published in 1949, Beauvoir shows how pubescent girls begin to garner men's attention and resultingly start to experience their bodies as "foreign" to them. That is, they begin to see themselves from the outside, through the eyes of men, who, without compunction, gaze at or comment on their body. This phenomenon, usually referred to as "sexual objectification," will be our focus in this chapter. We'll also ask whether all objectification is sexual or whether there are variations on the experience, and we'll consider how dieting to fit the thinness ideal affects teens. Our central question will be: *What's it like to come of age in a society obsessed with girls' bodies?*

What's Sexual Objectification? And How Does It Affect Us as Teens?

Since it's a common phenomenon and rite of passage for young women, you might already be familiar with the expression "sexual objectification." But you may not know that this phenomenon hinges on a philosophical distinction made in the twentieth century between *body-as-object* and *body-as-subject*. Philosophers who made this distinction belonged to a school called phenomenology. One thing that made phenomenologists unique is that they didn't want to get caught up in endless philosophical debates ("What's the connection between mind and matter?" "Can we prove the existence of God or not?" and so on). Instead, they were interested in *describing* how we experience ourselves and the world. In 1932, at a French cocktail bar, the philosopher Raymond Aron went so far as to tell Beauvoir and her lifelong companion, Jean-Paul Sartre, "If you are a phenomenologist, you can talk about this cocktail and make philosophy out of it!"[1]

This is the type of project Beauvoir is up to in *The Second Sex*. Beauvoir lived through an upheaval in women's lives around the globe—women were gaining the right to vote and entering the workforce in greater numbers, among other changes. Born at the turn of the twentieth century, she had to wait well into adulthood to be granted voting rights, as France did not allow women to vote until 1944. *The Second Sex*, published just a few years later, grapples with these changes. Beauvoir begins by refuting theories that seem astounding today—for example, that a woman is like a giant ovum (i.e., passive), and as a result, belongs at home! After criticizing these and other unsavory views, she develops a "phenomenology" of girls' and women's experiences. Specifically, she describes how girls and women relate to their bodies from childhood through old age. If you've heard the sentence "One is not born, but rather becomes, a woman," that's Beauvoir![2] This famous line invites us to look at how one becomes a woman, in particular, through the eyes of a teenage girl as she realizes that girls are viewed by men differently as they grow older.

But back to body-as-object vs. body-as-subject—which is a crucial distinction in the background of Beauvoir's theories and those of other phenomenologists. When we conceive of the body as an object, we're usually thinking about its physical properties, like its weight or height. Your doctor takes this type of perspective on your body when they take your measurements during a medical examination. We also consider bodies as objects when we judge them to be beautiful or not. This is what philosophers would call an "evaluative" stance. Basically, we're judging whether our body lives up to beauty standards: ugly vs. pretty, bad skin vs. good skin, and so on.

If, however, we approach the idea of the body as a subject, we're considering different kinds of properties—how we experience the world. For example, it's through our senses, like sight and hearing, that we access the world subjectively. We also act on things by using our body (throwing a ball), and other things also act on us (bumping our shin). And we experience pleasure and pain through our body.

The body-as-object vs. body-as-subject distinction is important because we often focus on how our body appears to others (is it a good-looking object?), and we forget that it's thanks to our body that we can see the sun rise over the water, that we can tug on our dog's leash when she's being stubborn, or that we can enjoy a nice cup of coffee while writing. What do we lose when we fixate on bodies' appearances as objects? What possibilities do we neglect when we forget that our bodies are also subjects? A lot! That's what I'll try to show throughout this book.

So what does "sexual objectification" even mean? Feminist philosophers have debated how to define the term for decades since Beauvoir, and the literature continues to grow with newer descriptors of the phenomenon. To keep things manageable, we'll home in on two features of objectification that are emblematic of girls' and women's experiences: the *reduction of a person to their body* and *instrumentalization*. Note that not all objectification takes this form. And for some philosophers, it's even pointless to try to nail down all the characteristics of objectification! Still, it's useful to have some vocabulary for the kinds of experiences that shape our attitudes toward ourselves and our bodies.

Let's start with the idea of reduction. What does it mean to *reduce a person to their body*? Quite simply, it amounts to "treating someone as primarily to be identified with their body or body parts," says feminist thinker Rae Langton, who developed the idea in the 2000s.[3] When a man ogles a girl's breasts or yells "nice ass," he has reduced her to one of her body parts and its appearance. In doing so, he neglects her subjectivity—the fact that she's experiencing the world and acting on it. Feminists use the term "the male gaze" to capture experiences like these. This expression refers to a reductive way of seeing and understanding girls and women, from the point of view of heterosexual men. Perceiving girls and women in this way, first discussed by Laura Mulvey in "Visual Pleasure and Narrative Cinema," sexualizes them and makes them appear passive.[4]

The *instrumentalization*, first depicted by philosopher Martha Nussbaum in the 1990s, happens when we treat a person merely as a tool, as opposed to what philosophers call an "agent."[5] Acting as though someone were a tool amounts to using them to serve your own ends without regard for theirs. By contrast, respecting someone's agency means you're considering the goal they set for themselves. Although you might disagree with another person's course of action, you can respect that person by engaging them in dialogue to convince them to pursue other ends, or by distancing yourself from them. Slavery is a clear-cut case of instrumentalization. Unlike a paid farm laborer (assuming the wages are fair and labor conditions acceptable), a slave has no choice but to carry out the work required of them. They can't decide *whether* to do the farm labor or *how* to engage in it. Given this situation, the slave owner can treat them as a disposable tool, replaceable by another slave or even by a machine.

Regarding girls' experiences, the sexual culture of many college campuses is one place where we see objectification take the form of instrumentalization. As Beauvoir scholar Nancy Bauer documents in her exploration of hook-up culture in the 2010s, college-age men have sometimes expected unreciprocated oral sex from women at parties.[6] The women who participate in this culture are treated as little more than sex objects. Although they can refuse to perform oral sex and, as Bauer points out, may derive a sense of agency from this possibility, there is still an asymmetry in these exchanges. To her knowledge (and mine!), college campuses where men are pressured to perform oral sex on random women don't exist. It's worth emphasizing that Bauer doesn't criticize the sexual freedom involved in hooking up. Instead, she worries that the playing field between men and women is uneven in these encounters. Men who rack up sexual encounters outside committed relationships are considered "players" and admired for their sexual prowess, but their female counterparts often end up labeled "whores" and censured for their promiscuity. Instead of analyzing these phenomena and double standards in detail here, I want to keep them in mind as examples of teenage girls being confronted with the idea that they are mere sex objects in the eyes of boys. This objectification makes girls understand their bodies as solely physical and encourages them to chase physical ideals, like thinness.

Bauer's research reveals that girls' objectification is very much alive today and isn't just a topic for Beauvoir. Her writings dovetail with the psychologist Renee Engeln's discussion of the objectification of girls and women today. In *Beauty Sick*, she provides statistics to help us quantify the phenomenon analyzed by feminists. For example, citing a study of five thousand US women, Engeln says, "85 percent of women reported first experiencing street harassment before the age of seventeen."[7] This statistic was corroborated in a follow-up study gathering data across twenty-one other countries, she notes.

How does sexual objectification affect us in our teens? *Self-objectification* is the answer. According to Beauvoir, before puberty, girls largely experience their bodies as the medium through which they express their intentions and perceive the world. They consider their bodies to be *subjects,* without feeling reduced to being a body with objective attributes. For example, a girl running competitively with her classmates does not explicitly attend to her legs. She has what philosophers call a "transparent" relationship to her body. The focus of her attention is on the finish line—not the shape of her legs. Her body recedes from her consciousness to give way to her perception of the finish line. But this situation changes at puberty. Once girls attract the male gaze, they feel their bodies as the objects of others' attraction or disapproval. Whether we're talking about catcalling on a street corner or comments on social media, girls filter their experience of their bodies through this gaze. Commenting on Beauvoir's analysis, philosopher Kristin Zeiler notes that a woman "comes to identify herself with her body as an object because of how she has learned to see herself, through and in interactions with others."[8]

Like Beauvoir, Engeln describes how seeing oneself as an object in the eyes of others lays the ground for self-objectification: "The more you are objectified, the more your body will begin to feel like a performance piece instead of the home in which you live."[9] This statement raises an issue that plagues girls. What kind of performance do I need to put on? Or to use more colloquial terms, *How can I look my best?* Self-objectification leads to what Engeln calls "beauty sickness"—the pain girls experience with body image and beauty standards. They feel pressured to look pretty, all the while suffering the harms of contorting themselves into shapes desirable to others. When this happens, girls' attention becomes divided between how their bodies feel from the inside and how they look to others.

Having your attention divided in this way creates real-world consequences that often go unnoticed. Engeln mentions the findings of the "bathing suit studies," where, after trying on a bathing suit, women tended to perform more poorly on a math exam; in another case, test subjects experienced body shame even ten minutes after dressing again. "The problem with having your body on your mind," she explains, "is that it takes your mind away from other things."[10] And unfortunately, this self-consciousness doesn't necessarily ebb with age. In the next chapter, I'll portray how beauty culture leads to a split sense of self in adults, too.

Yikes! Now I Can't Stand Being Looked At!

Even if they've already internalized some beauty standards, including today's ideal of slenderness, girls will likely have fewer body image issues in their early years. But as I noted earlier, children may already struggle with body dissatisfaction before puberty. It could start when parents shame a child, or schoolmates bully her because of her weight. Sexual objectification, however, ramps up at puberty, and until then, a girl may not feel the force of the male gaze.

Sexual objectification and its sidekick, self-objectification, trigger shame. Philosophers define shame as an emotion originating in real or perceived transgressions. Discussions of shame go as far back as the ancient Greek thinker Aristotle, who characterized shame as a "fear of disrepute."[11] With this ancient comment in mind, let's zoom ahead to present-day theories. The contemporary philosopher Luna Dolezal writes that shame is "an emotion of self-assessment which causes the subject to feel anxiety at the thought of how he or she is seen and judged by others."[12] She calls shame a "self-conscious emotion" since it entails either the concrete or imagined presence of other people.[13] *Body shame*, specifically, is an emotion directed at the "seen body"—namely, the body as it's perceived (or imagined to be perceived) in the eyes of others, Dolezal says. In the case of body shame, we may not feel something as lofty as Aristotle's "fear of disrepute," but we do fear criticism, whether it's a piercing glance at or a catty remark about our body.

Is experiencing shame a bad thing? According to Dolezal, sometimes yes, but also sometimes no. She distinguishes between benign forms of shame and detrimental ones. Cases of benign shame (for example, knocking over your drink on a first date) typically fall under the scope of what we would call "embarrassment." We run into problems when shame becomes *limiting*. Such shame "can be restricting and must be overcome for life to have the possibility of dignity and fulfillment," Dolezal writes.[14] She gives the example of a woman who is so ashamed of the shape of her nose that it prevents her from having a normal conversation. Limiting body shame overwhelms us and stands in the way of our everyday activities.

As an example of limiting body shame at puberty, consider Beauvoir again. In *The Second Sex*, she mentions one girl's experience: "For two years I wore capes to hide my chest, I was so ashamed of it."[15] Even today, feeling this shame is common. Like this girl, I also hid my chest for a year and refused to undress in front of anyone, simply because

I was developing breasts. By the time I first acquired a bra, though, that shame would dissipate. According to the feminist philosopher Iris Marion Young, what's worse is that girls often connect the changes in their bodies, such as menstruation and breast development, with the unwanted attention they receive from men.[16] Their physical changes, instead of being sources of pride, become ones of shame. Engeln's research in psychology echoes Beauvoir's account. "By age thirteen, body shame is common in girls, and girls already report significantly more body shame than boys," Engeln writes.[17] So let's recognize how important it is for our flourishing to come to terms with these significant moments in our lives. And a starting point is to acknowledge them.

Even if their bodies live up to conventional beauty standards, girls can be harmed by self-objectification because it incentivizes them to focus on their bodies at the expense of other aspects of their selves. A young girl may see her body as a source of power—for example, her legs propel her during games and sports. But as time goes by, she learns that her legs are objects *for* others—things whose appearance needs to be controlled (for example, by shaving them). Of course, the same goes for other parts of her body. In fact, the feminist Sandra Bartky depicts *fragmentation* as a hallmark of girls' and women's experiences of their bodies.[18] We try to micromanage the appearance of each body part, as if it were a separate entity. Eyebrows need tweezing, legs need shaving, hair needs styling, and maybe coloring. Our face must have one type of moisturizer, while the rest of our body must have another. Still, you might reply, thinking of our legs as a source of power sounds like fragmentation! But it is not fragmentation—the girl I'm inviting you to imagine is using her legs to express herself, not to objectify herself. Also, when delighting in the power of her legs, she is a whole person, not just her legs. She uses them to get her entire body from one place to another: her body as subject, taking action.

Objectification, by contrast, shuts down such a holistic experience of the body. To return to Beauvoir's example, when a random man comments on the "fat calves" of a pubescent girl, he has isolated that part of her body from the rest of her. Her calves are for him (to appraise). *Not* for her (to enjoy). What's more, he doesn't want to connect them to any other part of her body (or self). The girl's calves are just there—up for his dissecting gaze.

Is All Objectification Sexual? What About "Beauty Objectification"?

For a long time, feminists equated objectification with *sexual* objectification. But the winds are changing. In recent years, some philosophers have argued that the pressure to look beautiful has ramped up so much that we should talk of "beauty objectification." Let's dive into this concept.

Heather Widdows, whose work I mentioned in chapter 1, suggests that "beauty objectification is not necessarily sexual if it does not carry an implied sexual threat and can be distanced from sexual desire."[19] Basically, when we evaluate ourselves and others in terms of beauty standards, we're treating our bodies as objects without a sexual intent in our gaze. Take a common case. When we judge a woman for "letting herself go" because she has gained weight, we're considering her body as an object. And when that woman experiences shame, she's also treating her body like an object. There's a discrepancy between the reality of her body and the body she aspires to have. Just as we might be disappointed when the furniture we were eyeing online doesn't look as good when it arrives, so too we feel ashamed when our body doesn't look "good enough." In this case, there's no suggestion that the woman who put on weight is being treated as a "sex object" or that she experiences herself as such.

Still, there are other ways of exploring examples like these, and different conclusions to reach. After all, don't our beauty standards derive from judgments of sexual attractiveness? Widdows responds that even if sexual desire shapes our beauty standards, our sexual preferences aren't the *only* factor in objectifying ourselves and others. For example, heterosexual men have been reported to idealize a slightly larger body size in women than women do in themselves. So the woman who has added only a few pounds may remain sexually attractive to men, yet other women may still judge her, or she may judge herself, for not being as thin as she used to be. This conclusion reveals that there's more to her objectification or self-objectification than mere sexual attractiveness. Further, if we look at girls' and women's lived experiences—specifically, how we feel about our appearance—there may not be any sexual desire "in play."[20] When we look in the mirror, the male gaze may not factor in our relationship to our body. When I caught my father looking at my stomach as a teen, I did not feel any sexual threat—only the sense that my body wasn't "good enough" and that, to avoid this shame, I needed to look as thin as possible. Any added pounds would threaten my appearance—not my sexual attractiveness.

Does the idea of beauty objectification imply that any focus on our appearance amounts to self-objectification? Does a man who worries about his abs objectify himself by Widdows's standards? In the feminist tradition, the concept of objectification originated in descriptions of girls' and women's experiences of the male gaze. It wouldn't have made sense to speak of women objectifying men or men objectifying themselves. That kind of analysis would have deprived the concept of objectification of its feminist "oomph," to draw on other work by Nancy Bauer.[21] So it's more helpful to think of beauty objectification as a later-born sibling of the sexual objectification at the heart of feminist thinking. Beauty objectification affects us all, while the original concept of sexual objectification was about how heterosexual men viewed women.

Another question you might have about objectification arises from everyday examples where it looks like we're treating others as objects. When I yank on my friend's arm as a car is threatening to plow into her, am I objectifying her? You could say that, in a limited sense, she's being treated like an object (a very fragile one!). I do not reflect on her personal agency but make a snap decision to save her life. That's not what I mean by objectification. Not any instance of "treating" someone as an object counts. Contemporary feminists and I fret over the reductive and shame-inducing ways people of all genders relate to their bodies because of demanding beauty standards. Our body anxiety is the problem. So let's look at it carefully as well as fearlessly, and gather our best resources to overcome it.

Who Teaches Us to Hate Our Bodies?

As I mentioned earlier, psychological research usually identifies three factors in the genesis of body satisfaction or dissatisfaction: family, peers, and media. At this point, let's consider each factor's impact.

First, the family environment. When searching for the causes of girls' dissatisfaction with their bodies, researchers have historically focused on body image in female family members, concluding that girls absorb the norms of thinness from the other women in their lives. In *Beauty Sick*, Engeln depicts how girls pick up on conversations among older women in their family (for example, their mothers or sisters). Thanks to these women, girls learn to hate their bodies. "Fat talk" is a prime example of this. As Engeln explains, such talk amounts to disparaging ourselves for not being thin enough. Stomach rolls, large thighs, or arm flab—all are fodder for fat talk.[22]

Although the focus has been on the influence of mothers and other female family members, there's evidence that fathers play a role in girls' body satisfaction or dissatisfaction as well. In an article from the journal *Body Image*, researchers Jaclyn Siegel, Virginia Ramseyer Winter, and Mackenzie Cook discuss the positive influence of conversations between fathers and daughters on girls' body image. Their findings indicate that fathers "recognize the importance of these conversations but face numerous challenges to having these critical discussions," and that it's important for them "to support their daughters' skills, strengths, and talents, and avoid stigmatizing language around weight and body size."[23]

Second, just as family members contribute to shaping our body image, so too do the conversations we have with our peers. Fat talk is a classic topic among teenage girls. It lays the ground for the harmful strategies girls use to manage their weight. For instance, girls often learn binge/purge behaviors from each other and may even engage in them together. I know this from conversations I have had with adults reflecting on their teenage years.

Third, traditional (and now social) media impacts girls' body image. Take the effects of publications like *Seventeen* on teenage girls. "An analysis of over ten years of *Seventeen* magazine revealed a focus on the creation of 'body problems' in the minds of girls," Engeln writes, "a laundry list of body areas that need to be managed and nightmare scenarios about bodies gone wrong. . . Long legs good. Short legs bad. Flat belly good. Belly rolls bad."[24] What is worse is the hypocrisy—such media outlets often "also contain articles encouraging girls and women to 'empower' themselves by fighting against the very same body ideals promoted in their pages."[25] Similar conclusions apply to social media. According to 2025 Pew Research Center data, most teens visit Instagram, Snapchat, YouTube, and TikTok daily, with one in five teens going so far as to say that they're on the latter two platforms "almost constantly."[26] Given the messaging found online and on social media apps, it's easy to imagine how the staggering amount of time teens spend there would translate to body image issues.

Online platforms represent the same narrow ideals already featured in traditional media. But they also create communities focused on weight loss, such as the thinspo sites of the 2010s, or the networks based on hashtags like #SkinnyTok in the 2020s (we'll talk more about these in chapter 4). These communities are dangerous because they present, as Engeln puts it, "a predictable series of emaciated-looking models and inspirational quotes aimed at promoting starvation diets."[27] They also incentivize an excessive focus on the body and use body-shaming language. Researcher Sarah Grogan surveys how magazine exposure, images of women's bodies on the internet, and social media all drive body dissatisfaction in girls. Tweens and teens who used social networking sites, Grogan reports, "scored significantly higher on body concern than non-users, suggesting that internalization of thin ideals mediates the relationship between social media exposure and body concerns."[28] So if you didn't grow up with Instagram or TikTok, consider yourself lucky! That said, even though I was fortunate enough to have grown up before social media and only had access to the photoshopped women of glossy magazines, their content would leave as indelible a mark as my father's glance at my stomach when I wore my first crop top.

Why Is Teen Dieting So Worrisome?

According to a 2023 literature review published in *Adolescents*, disordered eating behaviors—which are abnormal eating behaviors that don't meet the criteria for a diagnosis of "eating disorder"—are widespread, affecting up to 22 percent of children and adolescents.[29] Parents are one source of influence in the development of these behaviors. Although the authors caution that more research is needed to determine the full effects of parental behavior on teenagers, they acknowledge that in their own clinical experience with adolescents with eating disorders and disordered eating behaviors, "many parents act as models of disordered eating behaviors for their children, and even if this is not the main risk factor for developing an ED, it could be considered an important one."[30] The picture concerning peer effects is more complicated; studies highlight that teens who engage in disordered eating tend to isolate, which suggests that friends may not encourage extreme behaviors in the long term.[31] Teenagers turning to "pro-ana" ("pro-anorexia") or "pro-mia" ("pro-bulimia") websites indicates that they may find encouragement and resources there that fuel eating disorders. But researchers note that peers can also be found in online communities that offer help with eating disorders.[32] We'll learn more about the power of communities of resistance in part 2, but for the moment let's underscore the strong effects that peers can have on each other. Finally, regarding the media, we see that many sources normalize dieting—from magazines at the supermarket checkout promoting the latest diet to sponsored ads that pop up on our social media feeds. Altogether, family members, peers, and media make dieting feel compulsory, and teens soak it all in.

I worry about these findings. Weight-loss dieting is a strong predictor for developing a full-fledged eating disorder—a connection that continues to be backed up by empirical research. A 2021 epidemiological review found that anorexia might affect up to 4 percent of women and up to 0.3 percent of men worldwide, and bulimia up to 3 percent of women and 1 percent of men, during their lifetime. The same study indicated that certain eating disorders, in particular anorexia, peak in the mid-teens, around age fifteen in girls, and that "several studies report a remarkable increase in the incidence of anorexia nervosa among girls aged 10–14 years."[33] Worse yet, eating disorders are considered some of the most lethal of psychiatric conditions. A 2013 study concluded that lifetime suicide attempts were significantly more common in women with any type of eating disorder, compared to women with no disordered eating.[34]

Just as we learn to objectify and critically judge our bodies, so too, we learn to diet. And when we diet, we put ourselves at risk for developing life-threatening illnesses.

At thirteen, I am a devotee of *Allure*. Every month, I look forward to picking up a copy from W.H. Smith, one of a handful of bookstores in Paris that carry English-language magazines and books. I pore over the tips on skin care and makeup and plan out wardrobes based on each season's new colors and fabrics. I learn about the best mascaras and how to put them on, as well as the concealers and blushes for my skin tone. Two years later, I fall for the extra sparkly look: I paint my nails a shimmering shade of brown and pair them with shiny green eyeshadow. More than anything, though, I dream of looking like the models posing on its bright and glossy covers. Perhaps I could even become one. I'm leggy and shooting up. People around me are starting to whisper that I should model.

One day, I'm curled up on my bedroom's white and blue chintz armchair. I've cupped my head in one hand and propped *Allure* on my lap. I'm reading about a famous runway model. She's six feet tall and weighs 130 pounds. I'm close to that height. Can I stay close to that weight?

130. I don't recall any more about what I read. Only the number—a number whose hold on me I took over twenty years to loosen.

Like teenage girls today, I absorbed beauty standards such as thinness and started to diet. During puberty, my family, peers, and media all made me feel the tyranny of slenderness. My experience differed from my peers' only because I started to feel pressure with the comments I received about modeling. I wanted to walk the runway. Yet I also wanted to spend hours learning the harp, studying calculus, and perfecting my German and Latin. In the next chapter, I'll explore this experience to show how girls and women come to feel divided between the demands of beauty and diet culture and those of their studies, careers, and relationships. These demands drain women of their time, money, and attention, and lead to a split sense of self. Deep down, many of us know that we should attend to other things besides a glowing complexion, perfect manicure, flat abdomen, or perky derrière. Yet our culture makes it so hard for us to block out the siren song of beauty . . .

3

Double Aims, Divided Aims

The Pleasures and Pains of Beauty Culture

> I must cream my body with a thousand creams, each designed to act against a different deficiency, oil it, pumice it, powder it, shave it, pluck it, depilate it, deodorize it, ooze it into just the right foundation, reduce it overall through Spartan dieting or else pump it up with silicone. I must try to resculpture it on the ideal through dozens of punishing exercises. If home measures fail, I must take it to the figure salon, or, inevitably, for those who can afford it, the plastic surgeon.
>
> —SANDRA BARTKY, "Narcissism, Femininity and Alienation"

"You should model."

At fifteen, I'm six feet tall. I've shot up from five feet seven in the previous two years. My body has the dimensions of a pubescent girl: narrow hips and no real boobs to speak of. Plus, I'm stick-thin. The perfect combination for modeling circa 2000. Only my family and classmates know that I'm a straight-A student. With strangers, I hear the refrain: "You should model." I walk into a restaurant, and the hostess will say, "You should model." I get a haircut, and the stylist will say, "You should model."

"You're too tall."

At sixteen, I send a couple of photos to French agencies. I've heard too many people encourage me to model to ignore the idea. Perhaps I could become a geneticist or a doctor, and a model, too. But when I send photos of myself in a bikini along with my measurements, I hear a new refrain: "You're too tall." Their cutoff is five feet ten. I shrug the rejections off.

"You should model."

At seventeen, I'm scouted in Harvard Square on Columbus Day. It's unseasonably warm, and I'm wearing a cutout top that's half yellow, half black lace. Maybe it's the outfit, or maybe it's my long, wild black hair that falls to my waist. A young man stops me. "You should model." He's a photographer and hands me the business card of a Boston-based modeling agency. I take the bait and attend a few appointments there. The agents first provide me with information about modeling. Afterward, a few of them swarm around me, and my hips, my waist, and my bust get measured. I feel like a prize cow at a state fair. I dislike this feeling, and I wonder whether it comes across to those sizing me up. Still, I spend a month shuttling between Cambridge and Boston before deciding not to sign an offer with them.

"You're too old."

At twenty-one, I give modeling one last shot. Why not make a little money to pad my time in graduate school? As I upload photos to the agency platforms in New York City, I'm conflicted. I'm not invested in modeling, and yet the "you should model" has never loosened its hold on me. I attend a few casting calls. This time, I hear a different summary judgment: "You have a great body, but you're too old." I'm hardly insulted. I know that agencies seek models they can represent for several years. Besides, I hate how the agents circle me to appraise my body. I'm too old to stand there like cattle.

THIS WAS MY BRIEF FORAY into modeling: I was intrigued by being invited to give it a try, but unwilling to put my heart into it, and ultimately too sensitive to allow myself to be sized up the way agents did, even if it was "just business" to them. But now I'm grateful for these experiences, since they provide a useful reference point for my own thinking about beauty and self-worth.

One of this chapter's main ideas is that beauty culture divides us. I felt this division most acutely over the years I considered modeling. I wanted both to be an exceptional student and to be an exemplar of feminine beauty. But these goals were not reconcilable, and in the end, only the first goal was really my own. During childhood and adolescence, my interests moved from paleontology to astronomy, then from veterinary science to genetics. I constructed dinosaur models, designed homes for earthworms, and blew up balloons with dots to represent the universe's expansion. Like many girls my age, I also played with Barbies. But other than that, nothing in my early youth pointed to a career in modeling or an obsession with beauty.

These experiences raise an important question, which is relevant to the thinness ideal and other aesthetic norms: *Why do we care so much about being beautiful?* Let's weigh the benefits beautification gives us and the downsides that come with equating our worth with our appearance.

Double Aims: Why Do We Care So Much About Being Beautiful?

In chapter 1, I mentioned that the philosopher Heather Widdows singles out slimness as one of the most pervasive beauty standards for women today. To better understand this standard's impact, we need to step back and investigate why beauty, in general, has such a strong claim on us.

According to Widdows, beauty has morphed into an *ethical ideal.* The pressure to look good has encroached to such an extent that it's become how we see ourselves as people, and opting out of beauty practices feels impossible for women, and for more men, too. "As we value beauty more and it becomes, for some, *the* most important value, we judge ourselves, our whole selves, as good or bad, failing or succeeding, as a person, according to the extent we attain the beauty ideal," Widdows says.[1] We're unlikely to say someone has "let themself go" when they drop their knitting hobby. But we'll use expressions like these regarding beauty. When we don't "work off" the "baby weight" or we let our locks go gray, many of us view ourselves *as failures.* To draw on the language of cognitive behavioral therapy, we magnify what is a local failure and make it into something global.

The beauty ideal is what Widdows calls a "collective framework," a set of behaviors and attitudes that affects a wide swath of people. Let's make this concrete. If my students fall asleep during a lecture, I may commiserate with colleagues. But failing as a teacher only matters to a small subset of the population. By contrast, beauty matters to many, many more people. We all know what a "bad hair day" is! But not everyone can relate to a "bad teaching day." That's what Widdows is getting at when she calls the beauty ideal a collective framework; it's "more dominant and powerful than a mere prudential or social norm." You may not act in your best interests when you skip a meeting as your company downsizes, or you might look awkward trying to eat sushi with a fork. But in all likelihood, people will judge you more harshly, and more often, for beauty "transgressions": showing up at work without makeup, lounging by the pool without removing "bikini line" hair, and so on.

What we call "beauty culture" is an expression of this ideal. The linguist Heather Spencer-Oatey defines culture as "a fuzzy set of basic assumptions and values, orientations to life, beliefs, policies, procedures and behavioral conventions that are shared by a group of people, and that influence (but do not determine) each member's behavior and his/her interpretations of the 'meaning' of other people's behavior."[2] To apply this definition to our topic, the actions and values we develop around beauty shape our personal choices day in and day out, as well as our relationships with others. We trudge to the gym in the hope of a more perfect body. We make catty comments about actresses who have put on weight. Although we could forgo these practices and judgments, they're so baked into our way of life that they form a culture.

In the same vein, "diet culture" refers to the assumptions that push us to want to lose weight and the actions we undertake to become leaner. We restrict food or change what we eat as part of this culture. We engage in "fat talk," that is, disparaging commentary on our weight or body size. Since the thinness ideal is so prevalent within today's dominant beauty norms, you could say that diet culture is just a subset of beauty culture. That said, you might respond that diet culture is something separate from beauty culture, since health concerns may motivate dieting. But as we saw in chapter 1, physical health is compatible with a wider range of body weights and shapes than we assume. Dieting feels compulsory for many women—regardless of their body size or health. Here you could draw a parallel between dieting and sexuality. Thinkers like Judith Butler have claimed that heterosexuality is compulsory in the sense that, in many times and places, we've treated being heterosexual as natural and considered any other behavior or desire deviant.[3] I'd say something similar about dieting today. We may think of trying to lose weight as natural, but it's often a disguised attempt to "look better." Or to circle back to Widdows's work, it's an attempt to "be better."

The notion that beauty is an "ethical ideal" or the claim that we partake in "beauty culture" or "diet culture" may seem abstract. But I hope the examples I've mentioned along the way help clarify these terms. At the heart of these theories is the idea that beauty guides our collective behavior. And it does so because we think it brings us benefits. Let's now have a closer look at what benefits we think we gain when we invest the time to conform to perceived ideals of beauty.

Quite simply, beauty work shields us from criticism and delivers certain concrete benefits, such as better romantic or career prospects. Or to put a different spin on this idea, "lookism," also called "appearance-based discrimination," is all too real. The psychologist Nancy Etcoff characterizes this type of discrimination as "one of the most pervasive but denied prejudices."[4] Let's consider this phenomenon in reference to thinness. As Kate Manne describes, "A wealth of research indicates that applicants with a higher BMI are less likely to be hired, compared with our thinner counterparts with the same profile and qualifications."[5] And as we discussed in chapter 1, fatphobia and anti-Black racism have long been intertwined. This suggests that appearance-based and race-based discrimination intersect. If we're biased—either explicitly or implicitly—to find Black bodies less attractive, then Black people will bear an even greater burden when it comes to lookism. And the same could be said about other groups stigmatized for their appearance—for example, those who have visible physical disabilities. It's also important to highlight that, compared to men, women bear the brunt of criticism when it comes to their looks. For example, a graying actor looks "dignified" as he ages. But the actress who fails to dye her hair just looks "frumpy." Putting these factors together, we see how racism, sexism, ableism, and ageism interact with lookism to make the lives of those already marginalized even worse.

Given the reality of lookism, a "makeover" or a "glow-up" promises tangible goods, such as a larger dating pool or more career options. Those who are a little outside the normal range will seek to transform their appearance to enhance their dating or job opportunities. But those who either lack the means or are too far outside our aesthetic norms will have fewer chances. The catch is this: The efforts of those who can "normalize" their appearance will dig a deeper divide between "the beautiful" and "the ugly," further disempowering those who cannot live up to standards of attractiveness.

Beyond these measurable social advantages, our physical transformations give us a more intangible sense that we're better, that we're doing better in life. If "beauty failures" increasingly feel like "global failures," then, conversely, successful physical enhancements become synonymous with success. Beautifying becomes self-improvement. Body becomes self.

Divided Aims: Can't We Be Pretty and Achieve Other Goals?

Beauty culture wields such influence over us that we struggle to ignore it. It promises rewards, like better job prospects, and a general sense of well-being. Still, we have other aims in life. And that's where we run into trouble. *Can we juggle beauty work and competing demands?*

The first way we feel split ourselves is concrete: We divide our time and money between beautification and other aims. Renee Engeln, whose research on "beauty sickness" we looked at in chapter 2, emphasizes the time and financial costs of beauty culture. She refers to an informal survey conducted by *Today*, according to which the average American woman spends fifty-five minutes a day getting ready, which adds up to two weeks per year.[6] The sheer number of articles on doing our makeup as quickly as possible makes one point clear: We're caught between competing demands on our time. Regarding money, the statistics also speak volumes. Engeln mentions that women do 85 percent of the spending on beauty products.[7] Given that cosmetics alone are a billion-dollar industry, this adds up to a lot of money! According to 2024 data, women in their thirties spent the most money, averaging $9,784 per year on beauty-related expenses.[8] By these numbers, if we saved $100 that we might spend monthly on beauty, after five years it would amount to the in-state tuition of a public college or university. These calculations suggest that we rob ourselves of other chances when we lavish money on beauty products. Now, if we add the cost of dieting plans—the diet industry is also worth billions—then the impact of beauty culture is even greater. Whether it's education or a different opportunity, the money we allocate to beauty could fund a lot of other things in our lives!

Of course, after reading this, you may want to wag your finger at those who spend their time and money on seemingly frivolous things. But as we've seen, looking good comes with benefits, like better dating or job prospects. This spending is imperative for acceptance at work and socially. And because our aesthetic standards are Eurocentric—that is, they favor physical features associated with whiteness—beauty work demands more of women of color. This is especially true for Black women, who, for example, may devote significant time and money to straightening their hair. According to one source, the hair-straightener market is estimated at $7 billion in 2025, and is projected to nearly double in the next ten years.[9] So we're not "sinking" our time and money into beauty, since we're also investing in social and financial security. That's where change gets tricky! Divesting of beauty and diet culture comes at a price. In *The Beauty Experiment*, Phoebe Baker Hyde documents her yearlong attempt to forgo cosmetics and other forms of beauty work.[10] She explains that she struggled to "keep up with appearances" when she ventured into important social events without any makeup on. She also agonized over what forms of body hair removal counted as beautification. Her experience speaks to the need to challenge appearance-based discrimination as a society. Otherwise, the costs of opting out will feel too weighty for one person to shoulder. (We'll get to collective action in part 2.)

The second way beauty splits us is by generating "double binds." To get a handle on this idea, let's turn to Marilyn Frye, a feminist philosopher writing in the 1980s. She describes double binds as "situations in which options are reduced to a very few and all of them expose one to penalty, censure or deprivation."[11] For example, when we label women who have active sex lives "slutty," we're making their sexuality into a bad thing. And when we call women who don't have sex "uptight," then we're also making their sexuality into a bad thing. Notably, Frye says that double binds are "one of the most characteristic and ubiquitous features of the world as experienced by oppressed people."[12]

We make similar judgments about the investment girls and women put into beauty. For example, according to Simone de Beauvoir, an intellectual will feel that she needs to appear feminine and will downplay her academic successes to avoid censure: "In becoming a bluestocking, a cerebral woman, she will either displease men in general or humiliate her husband or lover by being too dazzling a success. Not only will she apply herself all the more to appearing elegant and frivolous, but she will also hold herself back."[13] In other words, women will either live up to expectations that equate femininity with beauty or be dismissed by men.

But these issues aren't confined to Beauvoir's time. Sandra Bartky, a feminist philosopher writing in the 1980s and 1990s, mentions Dinah

Shore's words: "One of the many things men don't understand about women is the extent to which our self-esteem depends on how we feel we look at any given moment and how much we yearn for a compliment, at any age. If I had just won the Nobel Peace Prize but felt my hair looked awful, I would not be glowing with self-assurance when I entered the room."[14] This statement captures the tension so many of us embody from puberty onward. As a teenager, I hoped to become a scientist and even envisioned one day winning a Nobel Prize (I had tremendous ambition back then!). But like Shore, I, too, would have felt mortified if I'd walked into the ceremony not looking like someone who would be complimented for her beauty.

Today we've laid the label "bluestocking" to rest, but not the double standards about women's appearance. Take the example of women politicians. From the endless debates about Hillary Clinton's pantsuits to the comments about Senator Elizabeth Warren's appearance ("she dresses like a secretary"), they are wedged between two standards. The more feminine they appear, the less seriously they are taken, and the less feminine they appear, the easier it is to discount them as politicians at all. Women face the need to embody these enduring double aims. We must look attractive and excel at whatever other goals we have set for ourselves (or have had set for us). And even when the pressure to look beautiful conflicts with these goals, a compromise must be made, instead of abandoning beauty altogether. In my twenties, I felt this conflict at its highest pitch. I was caught between trying to excel as a philosophy student and restricting my food to look ultra-feminine.

This beauty/narcissism double bind is still alive and well. When we don't care about being attractive, we're dismissed (one bad thing!). That's the beauty part. But we're penalized for paying attention to our looks (another bad thing!). That's the narcissism part. Too much investment in our appearance marks women as lacking in intelligence or practical competence, and yet being unattractive would cast us out. Women are, as my mother would say, caught between a rock and a hard place.

When it comes to diet culture, we're also split. Working out excessively and only for the sake of weight loss has many downsides, including taking time away from friends or family. Even more extreme is the use of diet pills, which have potential health risks apart from the fact that they cost money. While we're still learning about the side effects of GLP-1s, they also cost us money we might spend on other activities or causes. This split is especially worrisome since dieting can pave the way for eating disorders. It also stands in the way of the very social changes that would transform our lives for the better. How much energy can we put into a political campaign or social activism if we're starving? The answer is little. In *The Beauty Myth*, Naomi Wolf argues that dieting is one way of controlling women: Deprive them of food, lower their energy levels, and they won't protest. How can you dumb down a woman who's fighting for her freedom? Starve her.

All in all, diet culture is a subtle form of oppression. As the sociologist Pierre Bourdieu would put it, dieting is a form of "symbolic violence." For him, symbolic violence differs from "overt violence" in that it involves a form of "complicity which is neither a passive submission to an external constraint nor a free adherence to values."[15] That may sound complicated, but his idea is simple. We don't subscribe to mainstream beauty standards because there's a gun to our head, but because we "choose" to participate in beauty culture. That choice seems "free." In reality, it's undertaken because of the enormous pressure we feel to look good. Plus, we don't have much say in which beauty standards dominate our culture. Why do we need to look *that* thin? Still, beautification is a choice. If we tie these different threads together, we see that we subject ourselves to punishing beauty standards because the penalties for failing to meet these standards are high. And the same goes for dieting. There is no jailer who cages us to deprive us of food. Instead, we do it to ourselves.

Can Beauty Be Redeemed? Considering Creativity and Power

I may sound anti-beauty, but that's not my point. I consider myself part of a group of feminists who claim that beautification has upsides.

One positive is the creativity some of us express in our cosmetic and fashion choices. In "The Fashion Model and the Beauty/Narcissism Double Bind," Cecilie Basberg Neumann tackles the beauty/narcissism double bind first depicted by Beauvoir. Neumann argues that modeling, a profession criticized by earlier feminists as superficial, has a creativity inherent in it. Based on interviews with models, she notes that the appeal of "coolness" and the "display of (self-) control" are part of the pleasures of modeling: "In high-fashion photography, this always requires exquisite display of bodily and emotional control and a certain kind of coolness, along with the fact that the model is supposed to look good and to be compliant regardless of her emotional state of being."[16] Although models may not choose their settings, makeup, or outfits during shoots, they may still experience themselves as co-creators of the images taken of them. They don't feel themselves to be mere "hangers" for clothing, a term sometimes used to portray the profession. Of course, this creative possibility hadn't occurred to me as I was being measured in the modeling agency. But it introduces the interesting possibility that even outside the world of photoshoots and catwalks, many of us can find pleasure in putting together an outfit and displaying ourselves to others. Naturally, not all dressing up and applying of makeup is fun, but Neumann's work suggests that we underestimate the combination of creativity and passion elicited by beauty work. Dismissing the creativity we embody when we doll up and dress up would fail to acknowledge "that beauty matters as a major source of creativity in human existence."[17]

Another reason we relish beautification is that it can make us feel powerful. In chapter 2 I mentioned Nancy Bauer's discussion of hook-up culture in the 2010s. There, she says that teenage girls performing oral sex can feel a sense of power over boys. As she puts it, "Being the object of the helpless desire of a boy you are about to fellate, especially when, at that moment, you're the only one around to fulfill it, can be—excuse the pun—a heady experience for a girl."[18] In these girls' experiences, sexual objectification becomes sexual empowerment because they're aware, instead of naïve, of the way they can use their beauty to shape sexual relationships. Commenting on Lady Gaga in another article, Bauer says she spins sexualized performances into "self-expression" and "self-empowerment." Gaga and the singers following in her footsteps are not just absorbing how to be feminine and desirable for men. Rather, they feel like agents in the very process of making themselves objects in the eyes of others. The paradox, though, is that to capture their gazes, they must nonetheless fit the mold. Bauer notes that Gaga is "pretty," "thin," and "well-proportioned."[19] Without these attributes, it's hard to see how she could magnetize us. And while we mortals may not have the star looks of a Lady Gaga or Sabrina Carpenter, we also get a kick out of being admired. It's nice to look beautiful in the mirror, and it's even nicer to have that beauty recognized. Whether it's the flirtatious gaze of a lover or the envious glance of another person, there's oh-so-much joy in wielding that power.

The points I've made here point to a much larger theme. Beautification is a cultural practice that allows us to communicate with others in our own time and place, and across generations. Wearing preppy vs. punk clothing broadcasts our values to others. Changes in fashion can signal political changes: Hippies grew their hair out in the 1960s and 1970s as a rebellion against the clean-cut looks of earlier decades. To neglect the cultural aspect of beauty work would be to fail to honor its cultural significance. So let's not be too quick to criticize the pursuit of beauty.

Redemption and the Promise of Community Pleasures

Besides being a source of creativity and power, beautification allows us to forge social connections. Heather Widdows mentions two ways that beauty culture creates social relationships. The first one is through *touch*. Having a manicure or haircut involves another's touch. I remember a summer spent studying alone in Berkeley, California, when I got a pedicure just to experience physical contact with someone else! I was surprised by my need to seek out touch. And I'll build upon the concept of touch in part 2, where I emphasize the power of sensual pleasure in resisting diet culture. In general, touch is an important part of beautification, whether it comes from someone else or the feel of our own clothes. In fact, Iris Marion Young, an earlier feminist thinker, claimed that *touching* our clothing could be a way of displacing the weight of the male gaze. Instead of seeing ourselves through a man's eyes, we can take joy in the weights and textures of the fabrics we wear.[20] Although Young was talking about resistance to sexual objectification, her ideas suggest that sight isn't the only sense involved in beautification. We can delight in the feel of our clothes. So too we can derive pleasure from the touch we experience when we're receiving beauty services.

The second way beauty nurtures us is by *bonding with others*. We commiserate with another woman applying eyeliner in a restroom. We catch up with our bestie at the manicurist's. We go shopping with our sister and gush over the most attractive outfits we discover. The philosopher Ann Cahill draws attention to the joys she experienced with her sisters preparing for her brother's wedding. To make sense of this phenomenon, she advocates distinguishing between "the process of beautification" and "its product."[21] She explains that the process lends women agency and helps them bond, while the product subjects them to scrutiny over which they have little control.[22] There's a difference between getting dressed up (often fun!) and the end result (not so much). It may be cool to get together with other "girls," put some makeup on, and shimmy into minidresses. But it's another thing to be looked at by the creepy guy at the club. So beauty can be a double-edged sword: It has its downsides, but it's also a way to nurture a sense of community.

We also may find a sense of kinship through online cultures celebrating bodies that fall outside the mainstream. In a 2023 article, philosopher Cheryl Frazier explores the resilience that members of fat communities develop when they deliberately choose clothes that are "unflattering" (per dominant norms) and share images of themselves in such clothing with other fat persons. The "Fuck Flattering!" movement drives home the idea that people of any weight should be able to "wear whatever the fuck they want."[23] For Frazier, beautifying oneself is a tool to "resist antifatness."[24] Here, bonding with others meets political combat. While such fights might entail stress or rejection from outsiders, they're also opportunities for beauty work to empower us.

In my view, we don't need to give up on beauty if we can define it to empower our creativity and improve our relations with others. As I've shown, we find joy in creating a sense of community from beautification. My concern is that many women feel that opting out of beauty practices seems impossible, even as they become increasingly demanding. Shaving our legs and underarms every few days may have long felt mandatory, but now we must add on a bikini wax or facial hair removal. An occasional pluck of eyebrow hair becomes a monthly threading regimen. And in sum, we've spent hours and hundreds of dollars on beauty work. We may feel guilty about all that time and money. Shouldn't we have spent time with friends or family, or saved money for a fun night out or a vacation? What's worse is that, at the end of the day, we rarely feel "good enough." As we'll see in chapter 4, clothing and beauty brands, and the expensive advertisers they hire to hawk their wares, want us to fail, repeatedly, to keep up with the latest fashions. Otherwise they wouldn't make a profit.

Still, the tide may be turning. In 2025, online influencer Melani Sanders climbed into the mainstream with her simple message: "We do not care."[25] Whether it's chin hair or a dress code, the "we do not care" attitude calls on women to drop the burdensome investment we have in caring for others and caring about what others think of us. Yet can we embrace this call to action regardless of age? I hope we can. But it will take a long time and a hard fight to get there. As I've emphasized using Widdows's philosophical account, beauty has morphed into an *ethical ideal.* This implies that we need *new* ideals if we're to loosen the grip of beauty on ourselves. And the same goes for diet culture. In my experience, the constraints of dieting eased thanks to the self-care practices I adopted when recovering from disordered eating. But beforehand, I struggled with a sense of hypocrisy about devoting mental energy to staying thin.

Since my undergrad days, I've committed to the feminist slogan "the personal is the political." In grad school, I draft a chapter on the genesis and dangers of the thigh gap obsession of the 2010s. I'm steeped in books on feminist philosophy for my research on gender, race, and embodiment. Three books—Young's *Throwing Like a Girl*, Bartky's *Femininity and Domination*, and Bordo's *Unbearable Weight*—teach me about the problems with excessive self-objectification and the patriarchal origins of our fixation on slenderness. As I work on that research chapter, I grow ashamed of my investment in the thinspo sites I continue to visit. How dare I criticize this obsession while I remain stuck in it? My "do as I say, not as I do" attitude makes me feel guilty, but I struggle to get a handle on my undereating on my own.

First, I try to apply Stoic ideas to my problems. The central idea behind Stoicism is that some things are in our control and others are not. Our intentions and actions are within our control. Fame, fortune, and property are not. I reason that my physical traits—including weight and size—are, at least partially, out of my control. I should only focus on what's in my control—eating well. Simple as that: My body's appearance is not up to me, but my actions are. It's time to put an end to the vain struggle to control my appearance.

I make a similar attempt with Spinoza's philosophy. Since reading his work in the second year of my PhD, I've admired his ideas about our emotions and the philosophy of life he builds off them. One of his thoughts is that perfecting ourselves means increasing our personal power. I dip into Spinoza's ideas as I continue to struggle with my sense of hypocrisy. Yet my perfectionism—being the perfect daughter, being perfect for modeling—drives me to want to look waifish and to eat as little as possible. How could doing that increase my power? Or is there a deeper meaning of perfection than living up to others' expectations? Does micromanaging my weight count as perfecting myself?

I reason that the perfectionism I've embodied since my teens is far removed from Spinoza's concept of perfection. Weighing 130 pounds or fitting into a size 2 has little to do with perfecting myself in his sense. The more I reflect on my predicament, the more I see that I'm not perfecting but destroying myself.

But neither Stoicism nor Spinoza is enough, on its own, to help. This is because I deal with myself through reason alone and can't find ways to put my ideas into practice. I don't implement any new habits to support my progress. All theory, no action. In my twenties, all my solo attempts at undoing my damaging eating habits fail.

4

The More Things Change, the More They Remain the Same

> Alienation . . . means the objectification or appropriation by one subject of another subject's body, action, or product of action, such that she or he does not recognize that objectification as having its origins in her or his experience. A subject's experience or action is alienated when it is defined or controlled by a subject who does not share one's assumptions or goals.
>
> —IRIS MARION YOUNG, "Pregnant Embodiment: Subjectivity and Alienation"

"Feet together, thighs apart."

I stand, move my feet together, and study my reflection in the full-length mirror. My bedroom's fluorescent light pierces through the dark blue outline of my jeans, highlighting the gap. "Feet together, thighs apart." I shuffle my jeans off to repeat the exercise. The same white light shines between my legs. "Feet together, thighs apart." I go through the exercise once more to ensure my hips aren't tilted too far forward, or else I would be cheating. What am I looking for?

I first discover the thigh gap while browsing thinspo websites at the age of twenty-five. I'm researching weight loss tips online. Thinspo comes to the rescue with its slogans ("skip dinner, wake up thinner") and its cruel imperatives ("do it for the thigh gap"). On these sites, I also find thinspirational photos of women above hashtags like #thighgap and #bikinibridge. I realize I have a bikini bridge, too: My abdomen is flat enough that a "bridge" could unite each hip bone. Yes, I'm already thin. But am I thin enough?

As I sift through the blogs, Tumblrs, and Pinterest boards, I'm reminded that I already know about thigh gaps. Just not under that name. As a teenager, I attended a Chanel and a Jean Paul Gaultier fashion show. All the models had thigh gaps. Whenever I recollect these shows, I can see one of the Gaultier models, clad all in black with the whiteness of the runway shining through the space between her pants. I already had a thigh gap back then, but not as pronounced. Since then I've yearned for a wide thigh gap and very thin legs. Only then will I be ethereal and beautiful like the runway models. Only then will I be the best version of myself. At least that is what one half of my divided self tells me.

AS SOMEONE who came of age in the late 1990s, I was sandwiched between two trends: "heroin chic" and "thinspo." And now, as I write about body image, I find myself researching videos under #SkinnyTok. Whether it's the jutting clavicles of models in glossy magazines from the 1990s, the thigh gap of thinspo sites in the 2010s, or the "legging legs" of TikTok in the 2020s, badges of thinness continue to be a fixation for many girls and women, fueled by fashion designers and online groups, social media and influencers. The more things change, the more they remain the same.

While body-positive activists have called on us to resist its allure, feminine slenderness has stuck as a beauty standard. I'll discuss the merits and shortcomings of the body positivity movement in the next chapter. But first let's have a closer look at the role of emblems of slimness. In this chapter, we'll dive into our fascination with the thigh gap and its sisters. I'll explore how this fascination stems from women's tendency to objectify themselves, the continued association of feminine beauty and thinness, and a visual culture that crystallizes this association. And despite backlash against trends such as heroin chic and thinspo, they continue to resurge. (As I write this chapter, "#SkinnyTok" is being banned, and the hashtag redirects to resources for help with eating disorders.) The roots of our focus on thinness are so deep that unless we dig into the weeds, we'll remain unable to accept our bodies. How can we stop a new version of these trends from sprouting up?

If this book's central aim is to inspire you to resist the thinness ideal, at the core of this chapter is a more specific question: *Why does thinness resurge repeatedly as a beauty standard?* Alongside, I'll explain how this slimness norm *alienates* us from our bodies. This crucial claim will take a while to unpack, but doing so is vital, since I ultimately want us to envision a world where we're not alienated from our bodies.

Selling Skinniness

In the beauty/narcissism double bind, women are encouraged to objectify themselves but are then reprimanded for focusing too much on their looks. But who encourages the objectification?

Writing in the 1980s, the feminist thinker Sandra Bartky highlights the workings of the *fashion-beauty complex*—the network of corporations that function to regulate bodily aesthetics. Whether they create beauty products or advertise them, these companies tell women that the body is a "task, an object in need of transformation."[1] But we can never fully master this task. For Bartky, images of beauty "remind us constantly that we fail to measure up."[2] Print and, today, social media instill in us a future-directed relation to our body: Transforming our body *will* fulfill us. As we saw in chapter 3, a makeover or glow-up will bring more than improved looks; beautification promises a "new you." Yet the billion-dollar beauty industry, long deemed "recession-proof," would collapse if we could ever attain its advertised ideals. Our wardrobe must reflect the latest looks. Wide-legged pants replace skinny jeans, distressed denims give way to relaxed fabrics, and so on. And our body must keep apace. Silhouettes fluctuate as we gain and lose weight. Taut skin sags and wrinkles (until the next round of Botox). Body hair grows back. Bodily wear-and-tear requires constant maintenance and repair until we live up—fleetingly—to reigning beauty standards. Or we stop caring. But this is a stance few of us have the luxury to adopt. Being pretty amounts to survival in a lookist society.

Our ongoing efforts to perfect our bodies, Bartky argues, are both *narcissistic* and *repressive*. They're narcissistic because we become obsessed with our looks. And they're repressive because we must always "discipline" our bodies to achieve, albeit temporarily, the right appearance. We punish ourselves. Yet Bartky points out that we also derive pleasure from this repression. She draws a comparison here between labor in capitalist economies and beauty work: Both are undertaken under pressure, and failing to meet demands has consequences for our very lives. But unlike an employee whose work goes unappreciated and would be ready to quit the moment they hit the jackpot, our beauty work feels rewarding. We derive a "narcissistic satisfaction" from it and become complicit with our own oppression.

If we take Bartky's analysis on board, we can see that our investment in symbols of slenderness is both narcissistic and repressive. To embody the look portrayed in images of the thigh gap or of skinny "legging legs," we must fixate on our physique. We stop caring *how* our legs are experienced from within—whether they feel strong from a workout or soft as we massage lotion into them. Instead, their *contours* matter. We compare our body to the selfies or reels posted online, as if trying to match a fabric swatch to another. But unlike the trials of coordinating materials, we can never achieve a satisfactory look for long. Weight is lost, then regained. And, as it did for me, dieting paves the path for disordered eating.

In the end, Bartky advocates a "non-repressive narcissism." We don't need to forgo beauty. Instead, we need to appreciate a wider range of bodies as attractive. She calls for "the release of our capacity to apprehend the beautiful from the narrow limits within which it is now confined."[3] This call to action anticipates the advocacy of body-positive activists, who want us to see that all bodies are beautiful. Today's activists are channeling the same idea when they call on companies to feature more diverse representations of beauty. This strategy is promising but has its weaknesses—we'll tackle body positivity head-on in the next chapter.

From Heroin Chic to Thinspo

Scholars like Timothy Hickman have said that contemporary imagery of toothpick-thin models with "hollow cheeks" and "panda eyes" is part of a longer trend, extending as far back as the nineteenth century, of "envisioning narcotic addiction."[4] What happened in the 1990s was a commercialization of this trend. These visuals fascinate us, Hickman says, because we have a "voyeuristic" need to see what happens when we let our desires take hold of us: "As we stare with fascination, revulsion or romantic longing at pictures of narcotic addicts trapped in their downward spiral, we ultimately confront our own obsessions."[5] Researcher Mary Rizzo claims that heroin chic arose both from the "upsurge" in heroin use in the 1990s and a return to "art and fashion photography of the 1970s, characterized by its realistic style and gritty subject matter."[6]

Regardless of the details, what's clear is that the 1990s glamorized waifish models in a way that challenged traditional pictures of beauty. Earlier images paired healthy-looking and pretty models with invitations to purchase whatever cosmetic, perfume, or clothing was on display, but this logic was inverted with heroin chic. Over time, concern over drug overdoses led critics of the trend to push for change in the industry. Hickman points out that after Davide Sorrenti, a photographer associated with the trend, died by overdose, "the fashion industry responded quickly. Partially out of guilt and sympathy, but also out of fear for its profits, fashion advertising changed course, seeking instead to promote a new, healthy image."[7] The model Kate Moss traded her sunken looks for a healthier image in her Calvin Klein ads. Yet thinness never went out of fashion, and thinspo took on the mantle of heroin chic.

The *online* visual culture that emerged in the 2010s is one of the main difference-makers between heroin chic and thinspo. During the heroin chic era, the fashion-beauty complex of the time lined runways and advertising campaigns with gaunt models. They also had advanced tools to accentuate thinness. For instance, some companies altered images of extremely thin models to erase the protrusion of their rib cages—leaving an ultra-slim silhouette that was (literally) impossible to attain without malnourishment.[8] But with the advent of social media, we took things into our own hands. Take the thigh gap fetish. When I first researched this trend in 2014, Googling "thigh gap" yielded a wealth of images, most of them taken by women involved in thinspo culture. The associated blogs and social media accounts differentiated between thinspo based on celebrities and "real thinspo"—that is, images of "real women" who had thigh gaps and bikini bridges.

Since the advent of smartphones, *we* have apps, such as Facetune, YouCam Perfect, and AirBrush, to alter images of ourselves and upload them to social media. And the use of such apps has blurred the traditional line between thinspo and "real thinspo" just mentioned. In fact, as I put it in my earlier research, "users . . . have reported that they forget what their faces and bodies look like through long-term use of them."[9] Our altered images become a currency on social media, generating likes and followers, thus upping the ante for those who don't live up to these images. In turn, we diet or turn to other weight-loss regimens, and in some cases start posting our own images, which generates a vicious cycle that marginalizes the few of us who don't opt into online beauty culture. "These technological advances skew our perception of what real bodies look like, thus widening the gap—no pun intended—between our actual bodily shapes and sizes and our perception of them."[10]

It's also worth stressing that thinspo sites echo the language associated with anorexia. In chapter 1, I mentioned feminist thinker Susan Bordo's idea that "garden-variety" dieting can lead to anorexia. According to her, one of the hallmarks of this eating disorder is the need for *control.* Anorectics feel a deep need to control their hunger.

This is what she calls "the control axis." Another feature of this disorder is a sense of being split between one's psyche and one's body: Efforts to control one's hunger are also efforts to control the body. Mind over matter. Bordo dubs this feature the "mind-body axis." The rhetoric of thinspo sites reflects these ideas. There, we find slogans like "keep calm and remember the thigh gap," "do it for the thigh gap," or "mind the thigh gap." These injunctions make it sound like the thigh gap is something outside of yourself, and you need to master yourself to attain it. You eat less because you keep your thigh gap *in mind.* This language makes visible the "control" and "mind-body" axes that Bordo thought characteristic of extreme dieting. I also want to highlight the crossover between thinspo and the more graphic and disturbing "pro-anorexia" or "pro-bulimia" sites that started cropping up online in the late 1990s. Both types of platforms have sought to offer support and encouragement for community members trying to whittle themselves down. Thinspo, however, puts on a more cheerful face and is more often publicly accessible.[11] Yet the downstream effects are similar: For some people, getting hooked on dieting foreshadows full-blown eating disorders.

Before getting into #SkinnyTok, let's pause to consider a seemingly more benign version of thinspo—namely, "fitspo." In this online subculture, fitness maxims like "strong is the new skinny" replaced the slogans of thinspo. Naturally, the visual appearances of those hooked on fitspo looked healthier. Yet as many have pointed out, the spirit of fitspo resembled that of thinspo. Both kinds of blogs featured photos of "real women" and ideal meals, descriptions of the exercises required to cultivate a certain physique, and motivational slogans. Thinspo cheered "thinner is winner," while fitspo declared "the harder the struggle, the more glorious the triumph." These communities also resembled each other in stigmatizing fat bodies. Thinspo asked, "Greasy fries or skinny thighs?" And fitspo echoed, "No ifs, ands, or jiggly butts." Moreover, fitspo, just like thinspo, promoted a culture of self-destruction. "Wanna get skinny?" thinspo said. "Fine. Then put down the fork, shut the trap, and starve, bitch, starve." And fitspo added, "When I exercise,

I wear all black. It's like a funeral for my fat." New beauty expectations cropped up. Instead of collarbones, it's chiseled arms. Instead of bikini bridges, hard abs. Fitspo did little but replicate the fatphobia of thinspo. Again, the more things change, the more they remain the same . . .

From Thinspo to #SkinnyTok

Concern that thinspo incentivized extreme dieting and set the stage for eating disorders led Instagram to ban #thinspo and its sisters in 2012. Meanwhile, body positivity positioned itself as an alternative to repressive beauty norms. Influencers from the "opposing" camp appeared online. Take Megan Jayne Crabbe (first known as @bodyposipanda), who preached body acceptance to her over one million Instagram followers. Around the same time, celebrities like the singer and songwriter Lizzo encouraged us to embrace self-love regardless of body size. Yet the tide has seemed to turn in the 2020s, with body positivity being eclipsed in an era defined by Ozempic and other GLP-1s.

To be sure, skinniness didn't go out of style between thinspo and the arrival of #SkinnyTok in 2025. Even before this hashtag rose to prominence, social media users continued to find other means to channel diet culture. Take #legginglegs, which surfaced in 2024. One of the main difference-makers between the 2010s and 2020s has been the popular uptake of GLP-1 medications for weight loss. Although Ozempic had been approved in the United States for treating diabetes in 2017, it wasn't until 2022, when celebrities began to tout its effectiveness for weight loss, that it and similar medications caught on. According to one source, TikTok videos tagged with #Ozempic got 2 million views in 2021—and 1.2 *billion* views in 2023.[12] Much like heroin chic in the 1990s, there's a synergy today between the use of substances that curb appetites and the glamorization of thinness. But unlike heroin chic, this tendency is driven by a prescribed medication as opposed to an illegal substance. What about the difference between thinspo and more recent currents? I think it's the sheer number of people on social media, paired with the thinner physiques that weight-loss meds make possible. In the early 2010s, thinspo content could be found on traditional blogs as well as on platforms like Pinterest and Instagram. However, with the advent of TikTok in 2016 and Instagram's growth from 500 million users to two billion users in the past decade, it's unsurprising that we now see a very powerful push for slim physiques.[13] The marketing of GLP-1s for weight loss is thriving on these changes in our social media landscape.

Another contemporary connection worth underlining is that between the 2020s "trad wife" movement and feminine slenderness. This movement is meant to inspire women to return to "traditional" gender roles, such as motherhood and homemaking. Naturally, this social shift has coincided with the rightward shift in political values in the United States since Donald Trump's first term as president. Since then, being a trad wife has become synonymous with social conservatism and a retrogressive conception of Christian faith—one that places women in the home and positions men as breadwinners. What's perhaps more surprising is the relationship between being a trad wife and slimness. Moderating one's appetite and religious aspirations have gone hand in hand for millennia. Yet some contemporary twists and turns deserve our attention. In the twentieth century, feminist thinkers went so far as to compare modern women's obsessiveness with thinness to religiosity. For instance, writing in the 1990s, Naomi Wolf explained that dieting became a new *altar* where women could sacrifice themselves in an increasingly secular society. Today, however, rather than restrictive eating serving as a replacement for religion, we see diet culture and religion colliding. As recent reporting has shown, the contemporary trad wife movement has picked up on these associations and made slenderness part of the package of what it means to be a good Christian woman.[14] The picture is even more complex if we read this change as unfolding on the backdrop of Ozempic: Some trad wife influencers go so far as to indict the use of weight-loss medication as "cheating." These criticisms imply that salvation can be found in dieting, and any "shortcut" to thinness is unworthy. Being skinny isn't good enough. Mastering one's hunger means mastering one's body, and mastering one's body means mastering oneself. "Pro-anorexia" and "pro-bulimia" websites from the 1990s onward personified anorexia and bulimia using the nicknames "Ana" and "Mia," while the thinspo sites of the 2010s told us to "do it" for a totem—the thigh gap or the bikini bridge. But now the trad wife pursues thinness in the name of a *higher power.*

What's So Bad About Striving for Slenderness?

Whether of a secular nature or tinged with religious undertones, our fixation on thinness seems problematic. But why? Is it because our obsessiveness leads some of us to disordered eating? Or is there a deeper concern that's relevant to us all?

One reason you might find badges like the thigh gap troublesome is that the thinness ideal is rooted in sexism. We can view its rise in the 1980s and '90s as a backlash to what's called the "second wave" of feminism of the 1960s and '70s: controlling our appetites as a way of controlling ourselves in a world that views women as a threat. A second reason you might worry about our focus on slenderness is that we women didn't craft this ideal; as Sandra Bartky claims, it's a creation of the fashion-beauty complex. If you follow her thinking, then you might decide that it's time that we take things into our own hands and develop our own (non-repressive) beauty standards.

These are solid reasons to reject heroin chic, thinspo, and #SkinnyTok. But there is another worry raised by their emblems of slenderness. My concern is that obsessing over them *alienates us from our bodies*. Let's unpack this claim.

In chapter 2, I reviewed the philosophical idea that the body is both a subject and an object. The body is a subject in the sense that it's our point of view on the world and the origin of our actions. It's thanks to my body that I'm seeing the screen in front of me and typing these words. Yet if someone comes along and bangs me on the head as I work on this chapter, I may pass out or even die. My body, an object, is caught in the chains of causes and effects that govern every part of the material world. As a physical thing, the body is also a being that others can view. People look at, touch, and judge our bodies. My doctor takes my pulse. In this case the evaluation may be neutral—a simple "check" of my cardiovascular system. But when it comes to beauty, bodies become too short, too fat, and so on. And when we internalize aesthetic standards, we often view our own body, our very self, as defective.

Experiencing the body overwhelmingly from the outside, as an object, leads to what feminist philosophers call *bodily alienation*. Philosophers use the term "alienation" to refer to situations where we become estranged from something that is naturally our own. For instance, if I'm alienated from my family members, that means that I don't have the relationship I once had with them. For feminists, bodily alienation happens as our body starts to feel foreign, strange to us. Alienation arises when someone else's interests influence how we relate to ourself. In the case of heroin chic, thinspo, and #SkinnyTok, it's the fashion-beauty complex, with all its punitive standards, that estranges us from our body. When we're alienated from our body, we start comparing it to other things. Most often, we compare our body to other human bodies and judge ourselves against whatever beauty standard is dominant. In chapter 9, we'll break down the idea of bodily alienation even further. For the moment, let's focus on this experience of alienation and its harms.

Bodily alienation interferes with our lives, and here's how it unfolds. When we experience our body as a subject, it tends to recede from our awareness. Mastering a bodily skill involves increasing seamlessness in how we coordinate our body parts and the objects we manipulate. To make this concrete, let's look at two examples. Imagine you're learning to play the piano. You start by tapping awkwardly on the piano keys and moving your fingers deliberately. But with time, your coordination improves, and you stop fixating on each finger. You begin focusing on the score or the emotions you're feeling as you play. You lose yourself in the performance of a piece. Or suppose you're a dancer learning a new set of choreographed moves. You acquire it first by slowly focusing on and executing each position. Over time these moves become a seamless flow integrated into your body. Whether it's manipulating piano keys or coordinating body parts, the same phenomenon is unfolding: Bodily movements become "incorporated." Just as we incorporate food into our physical bodies, so too we incorporate movements when they become second nature. There's a further important detail: Over time, the pianist or the dancer won't perform as well if their awareness stays focused on the specifics of how to make each movement. Once you're skilled at an activity, zeroing in on the minutiae can interfere with its performance. It's like being aware of the sound of your voice while speaking. The fluidity vanishes, and you begin to fumble your words.

When we become alienated from our bodies, the reverse of incorporation happens: We "excorporate" our bodily habits, to borrow a technical term from the philosopher Kristin Zeiler.[15] For example, when we laser in on our thighs in front of the mirror (as I did!), this body part comes to the forefront of our awareness. When we put on our jeans, rather than executing the required movements without any explicit awareness of our legs, we pause and become hyperaware of them. We obsess on them as objects, which interferes with our daily activities (and of course our self-image). We return to the mirror over and over again. We chant "feet together, thighs apart," just as our regular world falls apart. Whether or not our obsession with badges of slenderness gives way to a full-fledged eating disorder, we get in the way of ourselves. A once-natural relationship with the world is broken. We become broken.

The images that populate blogs and social media accounts dedicated to thinness mirror this breakdown. When I first came across thinspo in my personal life, I didn't think twice about the headless photos. But once I started combing through them for my academic research, I noticed that, in most images, heads were cropped or faces blurred. Of course, some women may want to protect their identity when they post pictures online. Regardless, the photos are framed so that the body *in its thinness* comes to the fore. Gone are smiles or other facial expressions. What's left is the body in its stark nakedness as an object. And that's the body that we interact with when we scroll through social media accounts glorifying thinness. We're reduced to our bodies, and what's worse is that we're reduced to fragments. Collages with collarbones, Pinterest boards with thigh gaps, and TikTok videos with legging legs—all reflect our dismembered selves.

Our obsessiveness with badges of thinness is borne of a view of women that diminishes rather than empowers them. It's propelled by fashion houses and advertisers rather than coming from ourselves. And it alienates us from our bodies. In part 2, we'll address ways to undo this alienation and to develop healthier ways of being in the world. For now, we'll keep our philosophical lenses on to analyze the harms of heroin chic, thinspo, and #SkinnyTok.

Beyond #SkinnyTok: What Can We Do Next?

In this chapter, I've zeroed in on symbols of slenderness from the 1990s to the 2020s. But the points I've made are relevant to the lean silhouettes of 1920s flappers or the waifish and leggy looks of the 1960s supermodel Twiggy, and they also extend to newer and newer fetishes. (I'm thinking of bony "yacht shoulders" as I write these words in 2025.) Does my analysis also apply to other markers of beauty, such as the fullness of lips, the appearance of eyelids, or the shape of eyebrows? One major difference between the iconic parts associated with thinness and other markers is that the cult of slenderness is more likely to create an unhealthy relationship with food or exercise than other infatuations. Having said this, I don't want to discount the danger of other fixations. People can obsess over their skin or hair to the point that their worries disrupt their lives. And people can go to great lengths with cosmetic surgery. So long as we live in the eyes of others, we'll feel the weight of their gazes. We'll want the approval of friends, family, or coworkers. And if we want to be publicly visible, we'll hunger for even more: gaining followers while avoiding bitter online trolls. Looking good is one way to grab the limelight.

As a professor working on body image, I'm sometimes faced with the question of how to distinguish harmless attention to one's appearance from excessive self-objectification, or how to recognize benign beauty practices from regimens run amok. The inability to care for oneself is one way to separate the harmless from the harmful. In my eyes, beauty work becomes excessive when it undermines our ability to engage in self-care. Here, I have in mind the slide I experienced from appearance-focused dieting to an eating disorder. But undermining one's very bodily existence isn't the only red flag. Conflicts in spending our money or time on other projects may also signal an unhealthy relationship to beauty. Of course, the issue is complex: Being attractive by conventional standards seems to promise specific tangible goods, like better career or dating prospects, as we saw in chapter 3. So it's not only a matter of beauty work vs. time with family or friends, or beauty spending vs. money on education or hobbies. Investing time and money in beauty work can also mean food on the table. We're doing what we can in a world that uses our appearance, especially body size, as a proxy for moral worth, economic value, and success. That's why it's hard to draw a clear line between the benign and the dangerous. That's also why pointing the finger at someone who's engaging in practices that seem extreme veers into victim-blaming. Before judging any individual for her actions, we need to look at the social circumstances that make her feel like she has no other resort but to do even more demanding beauty work.

As we'll see in the next chapter, the body positivity movement promised to change these circumstances—but its slogans, such as "all bodies are beautiful," only scratched the surface. To make true progress on the issue of body acceptance, we first need to challenge the importance of beauty in our lives, and also to challenge the symbolism behind markers of beauty.

Does being slender reflect self-discipline? Here I have in mind the rhetoric of social media today, and specifically comments like Geoffrey Miller's 2013 tweet, "Dear obese PhD applicants: if you didn't have the willpower to stop eating carbs, you won't have the willpower to do a dissertation #truth."[16] To be clear, I disagree with this sentiment. But even if there were a tight connection between thinness and self-discipline, we also need to ask ourselves why we value self-discipline so much. Is it because it makes us more employable in our economy? Where do we need to be more self-disciplined? And where might a more relaxed attitude be more valuable? You might have come across the slogan "A well-read woman is a dangerous creature." So is a well-fed one. And so is a well-rested one. Unless we fight for an entire society that wants well-read, well-nourished, and well-rested women, new forms of starvation for thinness will crop up. We'll continue checking the image in the mirror rather than facing the much deeper problems we can only solve with intelligence, collaboration, and truly empowered women.

"Body checking": the practice of checking one's body to evaluate its flaws. A term of art that would later be introduced by my eating disorder counselor. Thighs touching or not. Ribs protruding or not. Flab around the waist. Whether visual or tactile, the examination proceeds daily. Usually after my shower. But sometimes beforehand, when I undress. Why not be thorough?

I turn my body into an object whose appearance I appraise, as I would any other object. I check for scratches on my favorite paperweight, the yellow heart-shaped one that I'm looking at as I type. I check the dents created by knocking my furniture against my wall. It's the same principle, right?

Checking for scratches and dents on my prized possessions and property seems innocuous, even useful. I can avoid putting my paperweight on rough surfaces. I can repaint my wall. Doesn't it make sense to study my body from time to time? Does the difference between the two practices lie in the fact that my body is mine and the other objects are external?

That can't be the difference-maker. After all, I perform my monthly breast examination. If looking at or feeling my body like that is beneficial, then isn't it also good to body-check?

Bad faith: I'm lying to myself. The difference is patent. I inspect my breasts to ensure that I am in good health. I body-check to contort myself into a shape and size that defies nature.

Body checking leads to restricting food. I indulge in body checking for at least as long as I'm obsessed with the thigh gap. I know I'm underplaying the harms of my self-objectification and self-destructive behavior. How can I, as a philosopher, take thinspo seriously? How can I claim to be a feminist and indulge in a culture that's toxic to women? Facing these questions, and my own divided self, pains me in graduate school and my early years as a professor.

5

Body Positivity

A Revolution in Progress

> You have to act as if it were possible to radically transform the world. And you have to do it all the time.
>
> —ANGELA DAVIS[1]

It's the fall of 2018. I've been a philosophy professor for two years. Lunch at school is a candy bar brought from home or purchased from a vending machine. On my days off campus, it's two scrambled eggs, a few slices of avocado, and a spoonful of salsa. This would be a respectable lunch—if I didn't have it five times a week. The more worrisome part is dinner. This consists either of chocolate, a frozen Amy's meal, or a small bowl of cereal. I cannot remember the last time I cooked anything resembling a "real dinner"—that is, a warm, home-cooked meal with multiple ingredients.

The undereating that began with puberty continues, unchecked. As a result, except for a few months before my first hospitalization for depression, I'm always underweight. A few months after I leave the hospital, I start restricting, and my mood swings prevent me from caring for myself. The weight disappears, and after my second hospitalization, I continue to keep myself on a tight leash, so that it never creeps up again. I go from 139 pounds, my highest weight, back to 130.

I have been hovering around there for years. It's not a terribly low weight for my height, and I don't suffer any health consequences that I know of. I never feel sick enough for my problems to warrant medical attention. So I keep to my tiny meals. For years on end.

My reasoning is simple. If I enjoy food, I'll gain weight—the worst of all sins.

But by the time I seek counseling for depression, I know I should say something to my therapist, let's call her Chris. The dissonance between my feminist ideals and the reality of my body image and eating habits grows day by day. I know that it's wrong to bow to Thinness, that tyrant whose inflexible standards keep me and so many other women in check. Yet I don't know how I could live in anything but a thin body. Would anyone accept me?

I'm coy when Chris asks me about my eating habits, but the strain in my voice when I open up about my body-image issues must sound suspicious. I feign a smile when I tell her about the crop top incident and the years that I felt conflicted about the unsolicited advice I received to model. My tone sounds unconvincing to me, and surely to her, as well.

Chris recommends I see an eating disorder specialist at her practice. I hear the discordant notes in my voice during our weekly sessions and, hour by hour, in my inner monologue. The strain of lying to myself, and the realization that my new therapist sees it more clearly than I do, wounds me more than the dieting itself. I cannot ignore this tension anymore.

IN 2018, when I first considered seeking help for my restrictive eating, body positivity was in its heyday. The movement advocated accepting our bodies regardless of size, shape, skin tone, gender, and physical ability. Although it's often associated with online culture in the 2010s, it has a longer history, which we'll examine in this chapter, alongside criticisms of the movement. Once again we'll put on our philosophical lenses, this time to analyze the solution that body positivity proposed.

What Is Body Positivity? Where Did It Come From?

Body positivity grew from criticisms that had been voiced as far back as the 1960s, during the second wave of feminist activism. Feminists of the time challenged beauty standards they thought were too taxing. You might have the image of "bra-burning feminists" in mind. The truth is more complicated: Women protesting the 1968 Miss America pageant didn't, in fact, burn their bras. Instead, they ditched them in what they called a "Freedom Trash Can." (Better than creating a fire hazard!) Alongside, the fat acceptance movement was emerging. One key moment was the 1967 "fat-in" in Central Park. As the philosophers Cheryl Frazier and Nadia Mehdi explain in "Forgetting Fatness: The Violent Co-optation of the Body Positivity Movement," "Demonstrators burned diet books and pictures of the supermodel Twiggy and arrived carrying banners reading 'Fat Power' and 'Take a Fat Girl to Dinner.'"[2] These events laid the ground for the founding of the National Association to Advance Fat Acceptance in 1969. Fat activists wanted to bring awareness to discrimination against fat persons, especially within the medical profession. They also wanted to "undo fatphobia in schools, workplaces, and advertising."[3] In the next decade, other groups arose, such as the Fat Underground, known for its "Fat Liberation Manifesto" in 1973. The fat activism of the 1960s and 1970s called on society to provide equal care and respect for people regardless of weight or size.

Fast-forward to the 2000s. Following the debate over heroin chic, the fashion industry felt increasing pressure to project a "healthier" image and include more body types in its representations of beauty. Dove's Real Beauty campaign, which took off in 2004, pledged to change women's self-image by showing what "real beauty" looked like. Out were the haunting images of young, painfully thin models, and in came women of a greater range of body sizes and ages. As social media took off, users also leveraged digital platforms to voice messages of resistance to fatphobia and to champion more diverse representations of beauty. With more vocal calls for diversity, some fashion and cosmetic companies followed suit. Aerie lingerie later echoed "Don't

Change You! Change Your Bra!" As did Thirdlove with their "To Each Her Own" campaign for greater diversity. In the world of high-end fashion, some countries began to require models to meet weight thresholds to walk the runway.

Whereas earlier activism focused on weight stigma, body positivity came to encompass a wider range of concerns—the visibility of diverse gender expressions, skin tones, ages, and physical (dis)abilities came to the fore. The movement became less of a cause defending the dignity of fat persons and more of a framework for people to reject limiting beauty standards and embrace their bodies. Because of this shift, some people have questioned whether the movement serves the populations it was meant to support. In the 2020s, the surge in popularity of GLP-1s has introduced still new challenges to the body positivity movement, with many commentators announcing yet again that it is dead. But even before this period, body positivity encountered criticisms. Let's have a look at these, less in the spirit of a forensic examination, but rather to see what insights we can gain from the movement. Our mission in this book is to discover what's helpful and unhelpful in popular ideas about the body, so that we can reclaim beauty, health, and power for ourselves.

A Missed Revolution?

Rejecting body shame and the self-destructive behaviors that come from it sounds intuitive. And yet body positivity has faced significant objections. First, since the movement grew from fat activism, a major criticism was that it "glorified" obesity. The concern seems to be that body positivity neglects the medical problems associated with extra weight. That said, one possible response is to endorse weight-neutral health paradigms, such as Health at Every Size, which is founded on the idea that health and weight shouldn't be equated. Instead of trying to shame people into losing weight, this approach endorses a flexible and empowering approach to healthcare. The practitioners of this movement note that our health exists along a continuum, changing with time and circumstances for each person, and they emphasize the need for community care and mutual aid that "promote and create the conditions that support wellbeing, i.e., environmental care, clear air and water, equitable access to food, and more."[4] I think these suggestions are so important that I incorporate them in part 2 of this book. My recommendations also champion overcoming the body shame that diet culture breeds in us through a positive reassessment of our lives, grounded in self-compassion.

Now, back to our review of the cultural phenomenon of body positivity. Aside from worries about obesity, some people feel that body positivity has replaced unrealistic beauty standards with an unrealistic demand to "feel good" about your body. Because the fashion industry has only inched toward greater inclusivity, the "lag" means that we're supposed to love our bodies even if most representations of beauty are still out of our reach. Body positivity has also been charged with "toxic positivity"—the accusation that you must feel positive about something even if this betrays your genuine feelings. Positivity—whether related to the body or other topics—becomes "toxic" when it fails to recognize our natural wide range of emotions and makes us feel guilty for experiencing negative ones. *Why can't you turn your frown upside down? Why don't you just smile?* These questions reflect our society's discomfort with the darker side of the human condition. Toxic body positivity is unrealistic and disempowering. Kate Manne, whose work on fatphobia we considered in chapter 1, observes that body positivity doesn't seem to give us the space to define our own relationships to our bodies. Some of us may feel that our body falls short, or even "betrays" us, for example, in periods of illness.[5] So must we always feel enthusiastic about our body? Perhaps we can instead find some middle ground in the language of "body neutrality."

Before we jump into that, I want to mention another point: Body positivity may be too focused on beauty for its own good. An "all bodies are beautiful" ethos doesn't make room for those of us who are okay with not being attractive. This is a challenge that writer Mia Mingus voices in her speech "Moving Toward the Ugly: A Politic

Beyond Desirability." She says, "We must shift from a politic of desirability and beauty to a politic of ugly and magnificence. That moves us closer to bodies and movements that disrupt, dismantle, disturb."[6] Mingus is critical of the pressure that we *should* want to feel attractive. Indeed, a person who is not invested in their looks might value themself for other traits like their intelligence, moral virtue, artistic ability, or spirituality. The effort to make beauty more inclusive has been driving body positivity, and perhaps once we acknowledge that not everyone wants to look beautiful, the movement loses its impetus.

You might also wonder: Isn't the body more than an object to behold? Whether they're aware of the philosophical distinction or not, critics such as Mingus are appealing to the idea that the body is also a subject, as I described earlier. Our bodies get us around and allow us to encounter the surrounding world. By giving more weight to this aspect of embodiment, we value our bodies for what they can *do* as opposed to what they look like. Let's celebrate our physical capacities. Function over form![7] The criticism that body positivity is hyper-focused on appearance dovetails with the body neutrality movement. Body neutrality is often, though not necessarily, equated with learning to prize our bodies by engaging in movement or sports. Instead of trying to love the image of yourself, just smash the mirror! What's promising about this shift is that it honors the "subject" side of the body. But when this shift becomes all-or-nothing—just focus on your *physicality*—you might also worry that it's unrealistic in a world that gives so much importance to our *physiques*.

Another concern about body positivity is that it's become too commercialized—simply a marketing strategy to sell more goods. Do fashion companies *really* care about featuring more diverse models? In her research on communication in the 2010s, Jessica Cwynar-Horta writes that as body positivity gained popularity and influence, "corporations began commoditizing the body positive advocates and using their influence to push products, capitalizing on the movement."[8] She notes the Instagram collaboration between plus-size influencer Dani Adriana (then working under the username @chooselifewarrior) and NYX makeup. If you're on the more cynical end of the spectrum, you might go so far as to say that body positivity has become an arm of Sandra Bartky's "fashion-beauty complex," which Bartky defines as "a vast system of corporations—some of which manufacture products, others services and still others information, images and ideologies."[9] In the end, we have to acknowledge that despite its good intentions, body positivity has been used cleverly by marketers to sell clothing and cosmetics instead of helping people feel more at home in their bodies.

On a similar note, body positivity's mainstream marketing has been criticized for no longer serving the populations who created it. For example, the musician Lizzo, who was often associated with the movement, said in a 2021 interview, "Because now that body positivity has been co-opted by all bodies, and people are finally celebrating medium and small girls and people who occasionally get rolls, fat people are still getting the short end of this movement."[10] As I write this, in 2025, she has faced backlash for losing weight. Nevertheless, her earlier point remains: Because of the movement's expansion, it no longer seems to tackle the harms faced by fat communities. As Cheryl Frazier and Nadia Mehdi put it, body positivity "was designed to promote the radical acceptance of marginalized bodies. Proponents tried to shatter the perception that weight and health were conclusively linked and sought to remove the temptation to say that people needed to be healthy—and beautiful—to be worthy of dignity, respect and fair treatment."[11] Since body positivity was rooted in fat activism, they worry that including people who don't face weight stigma amounts to a "violent cooption."

These worries about body positivity are telling. The movement has been in serious need of repair. To mend it, we need to craft values that don't depend on glorifying any body type. We need to appreciate bodies for more than their image in the mirror, taking into consideration, for example, their capacities for movement and pleasure. And we also need to recognize that some people are more vulnerable—more likely to be dismissed, shamed, or discriminated against—because of their appearance. Body positivity, in a new guise, would be both individual by pushing for greater self-acceptance and political by forming coalitions across different marginalized communities.

What About Body Neutrality?

Because of the shortcomings of body positivity, a new rival came on the scene in the mid-2010s: body neutrality. One of the people credited with this idea is the eating disorder counselor Anne Poirier. "Body neutrality prioritizes the body's function, and what the body can do, rather than its appearance," she says. "You don't have to love or hate [your body]. You can feel neutral towards it."[12] As I noted earlier, some people have characterized body neutrality as a movement focusing on our physical abilities. But in general, as its name suggests, body neutrality means adopting neither a positive nor a negative view of one's body. The thought is to carve a middle ground between self-limiting body shame and toxic positivity. What's attractive about this neutrality idea is that it recognizes that you don't always feel great about yourself, and that telling yourself you love your body nonstop is counterproductive. There are merits to the idea that bodies are not just for appreciating from the outside. Valuing physical activity is one example of how to feel at home in your body. Still, body neutrality is not without its critics.

First, body neutrality's emphasis on physical capacities could be viewed as ableist. People who have raised this concern say that body positivity's rival excludes those for whom physical activities are a significant challenge. But it's very important not to assume that messaging such as "function over form" implies a new hierarchy in which people who are highly athletic are deemed to be more in their bodies than people who have challenges participating in conventional fitness or athletics.[13] I agree that this is an important concern, and it reminds us that messaging needs to be carefully scripted to refer to *your* body, whatever shape, size, or condition it may be in. We don't need to equate embracing movement with athleticism, and we don't need to equate being in your body with having a body that can run, pump iron, or do similar feats. Not at all. In fact, restorative physical activities, tailored to one's body as-is, offer a starting point for the kind of subjective experience that brings us power and awareness. So I encourage you to understand being in the body as a subject, and free of the standards of the beauty industry, as a different task for every human being.

Second, body neutrality can sound a bit underwhelming, or as Manne puts it more artfully, it can be "tinged with negativity."[14] Adopting a neutral attitude about one's body could seem bland at best, or unappealing at worst. But that's no reason to go rushing back to the arms of body positivity, either. Manne advocates a third way: body reflexivity. "A body is not something good or bad or neutral for people generally," she writes, "but rather something that may suit and work better or worse for its denizen—in other words, the person who inhabits it," since that person's "perspective on her body is the only one that matters."[15] That means that we get to decide what our body means to us. She positions her view within a "politics of autonomy that would vindicate the right to be fat, or trans, or nonbinary, or queer, or disabled."[16]

What's refreshing about Manne's proposal is that body reflexivity comes from within. You can be gleefully in love with your body or withhold any evaluation—whatever suits you. Likewise, the reasons for your attitude about your body are also up to you. One person may like their body for its beauty, another for its athletic prowess, a third for the pleasure it affords, and so on. And perhaps one person finds her shapely thighs attractive and values her arms for the things she can push and lift thanks to them. In part 2 I'll explore ideas for healing your relationship with your body that align with Manne's view.

The only difference between my position and Manne's is that I want to nudge us in the direction of self-love. For me, self-love doesn't imply toxic positivity. Just as loving someone else is compatible with a range of emotions—joy, pride, disappointment, anger, and so on—self-love can mean experiencing different emotions toward yourself. We may feel like our body lets us down at times, but, in the end, it is all that we have. This calls to mind a classic perspective dramatized by the existentialist Jean-Paul Sartre, who said that "I exist my body." By this, he meant that it is through our body that we engage with the world. And this brings us back to the existentialist challenge to be *in* our body and focus on the experience we have *through* our body.

Can We Revive the Revolution Body Positivity Promised?

I'd like to say a few words about what repairing our relationships with our bodies might look like—regardless of the trends within our society or large-scale events. I've suggested that a reformed body positivity movement should honor the body in all its aspects. My recommendations in part 2 include actions an individual can take, such as learning to eat mindfully or savoring the sensations of pleasure one's body affords. In my eyes, these endeavors originate in self-love. This kind of self-love doesn't require having gushy feelings about oneself (after all, each one of us has had days where we're none too satisfied with ourselves). Rather, it amounts to having a certain self-regard. Here it's useful to loop back to the philosopher Rousseau's account of self-love. He makes a distinction between self-love grounded in concern for one's own well-being (amour de soi) and self-esteem that's dependent on how others view us (amour propre). When we're filled with amour de soi, we undertake the actions that enable us to thrive, like getting adequate nutrition and rest. But when we're running only on amour propre, we're letting others' opinions determine our sense of worthiness.

Fashion trends (think heroin chic), medical upheavals (Ozempic), and even global threats (COVID-19 pandemic) shape how we interact with others and affect our body aesthetics. Slimness as a beauty standard hasn't gone out of fashion in decades, but its hold on us has tightened and loosened and tightened again. To weather these changes, we need to develop a strong sense of self-love—Rousseau's amour de soi. This form of self-love makes possible actions like eating enough or doing nurturing physical activities. The difficulty with cultivating this love is that we live in an unjust world that creates hierarchies between bodies: thin vs. fat, young vs. old, white vs. black or brown, able-bodied vs. disabled, cisgender vs. transgender, and so on. That's why just telling people to care for themselves will ring hollow in a world that doesn't care for them. From the sidelines, it's easy to encourage a person who's been judged for their weight to reject diet culture, but we must first recognize that we live in a society whose dominant messaging is that you are better and happier if you are thin or underweight. That person has a much harder time properly nourishing themself in such a society, since they're caught between their bodily needs and the thin/fat hierarchy that tells them to restrict their food intake.

Keep in mind that the work necessary to reform body positivity extends far beyond the individual. We need to tackle the "isms"—cissexism, racism, ageism, and ableism—that shape our society's beauty norms. Trying to uproot one's internalized antifatness will remain superficial if it only amounts to repeating "my body is beautiful" or "there are no bad bodies" in front of the mirror. A new version of body positivity must be political, informed by the need to address oppression in its many intersecting forms. In many cases, we may only feel secure in caring for ourselves once more people care for us. As the eating disorder expert Ann Saffi Biasetti says, some of us may not feel worthy of recovery until we truly hear the voices of others encouraging us to eat in life-affirming ways.[17] We can use this point to form our best response to the beauty industry, based on the self-care I promote. Since the impetus for us to care for ourselves can come both from within and from people around us, it can inspire us to be part of a community voicing love and encouragement. I intend this book to provide such encouragement. The true work of body positivity is to change the vicious cycle that elevates certain bodies at the expense of others into a virtuous one where self-care gives way to caring for others, and to further self-care.

In my experience, five years went by between the time I first encountered the feminist texts that pushed me to scrutinize my obsessiveness with being thin and my need to restrict food, and the beginning of my first round of eating disorder counseling. Telling myself I had a problem and coming up with half-hearted action plans hadn't yielded much. I yo-yoed in the land of "almost anorexia"—neither a weight that drew immediate concern nor one that would reflect a healthy relationship with food. It took the encouragement of my therapist at the time, Chris, for me to take the first step toward recovery.

In January 2019, after two months of conversations with Chris, I begin my first round of eating disorder counseling. I'm hopeful that I can quickly silence the tyrannical voice that has lectured me about my body and food for twenty years. Maybe I'll see the counselor for a few months.

My specialist, Dalit, is a tall and striking woman with jet-black hair pulled in a tight chignon. She looks to be my height, but as I follow her to her office, I notice her chunky wedges. She wears a billowy silk blouse and flowing pants. Her makeup is subtle, and her nails are perfectly manicured. The afternoon sunlight is streaming into the office we step into, and the couch I sit on is plush and white. It's a far cry from the predictable gray sofas that seem to occupy most other therapists' offices. The room would be uplifting, were I not here for a first counseling session.

"What brings you in?"

"I've had body image issues for a long time now. A long, long time. Since I was a teenager. I was encouraged to model. But I never did. I always get compliments on my body. I've been obsessed with being thin for years. Now it's gotten to me." My speech is pressured. By the time I reach the end of my complaints, I've contorted my arms and legs into tight knots.

"OK, now tell me. What do you eat daily? Do you cook? How often do you eat meals or snacks?"

I freeze. I don't know how to answer the question. I remember a boyfriend once asking me what I liked to eat and how he laughed when I answered "general food." I've learned my lesson from that moment, so I dabble in being vague. "I eat a variety of things. I love chocolate. I don't cook much . . ." That's about as far as I'm willing to go. Dalit must sense my discomfort and realize that it's too soon to push me. A smart move.

"How much do you think you weigh?"

"Maybe 127? 128?" The number is probably lower, but it feels safer to err on the side of overestimating it.

"Why don't you step on the scale? You can't look, though." She pauses and smiles. "I do blind weights. Not seeing the number will help you with your worries about your body. But I still need to weigh you to keep track of how you're doing in counseling."

I step on the scale. My heart starts racing. I'm panicked that I don't get to see the number. Relinquishing control feels even worse than facing the number itself. Her face is blank as she jots down the number at the top of a form. She must have perfected a poker face after years of counseling. I have no idea whether I guessed correctly.

After I settle back on the couch, she hands me a dark blue booklet, and we sit in silence as I leaf through it. It details exercises and expectations for eating disorder recovery. In a notebook, I will need to provide my responses to the exercises. For example, I'll have to describe role models in my life and whether I judge them on their appearance. Besides that, I'll need to record details of my daily food intake: what I ate, when I ate it, how full I felt beforehand, how full I felt afterward, and finally, whether I engaged in any "behaviors"—her euphemism, I take it, for disordered eating practices. She gives me the option between several small notebooks with various smiling faces and motivational slogans on their covers. I choose one with a pink, blue, and yellow background and a smiling French bulldog. Below the bulldog, the words "Be PAWsitive!"

6

Unbearable Weight

How the Pandemic Intensified Disordered Eating

Anorexia begins in, emerges out of, what is, in our time, a conventional feminine practice. In the course of that practice, for any number of individual reasons, the practice is pushed a little beyond the parameters of moderate dieting. The young woman discovers what it feels like to crave and want and need and yet, through the exercise of her own will, to triumph over that need. In the process, a new realm of meanings is discovered, a range of values and possibilities that Western culture has traditionally coded as "male" and rarely made available to women: an ethic and aesthetic of self-mastery and self-transcendence, expertise, and power over others through the example of superior will and control.

—SUSAN BORDO, *Unbearable Weight*

Besides the exercises in my Be PAWsitive! notebook, I need to take pictures of all the food I eat and upload them to a digital album I share with my counselor, Dalit.

I fill the first week of the album with photos of salads in small portions. At our next appointment, she takes her phone out to look at them. The slightest of frowns creeps over her forehead. She pauses.

"I'm curious about all the salads. Do you usually eat so many?"

"Not really." I feel my legs stiffen as I brace for her follow-up.

"I wonder, are you trying to be a model student?"

"Maybe."

Dalit is right, but I won't concede the truth. I'm too embarrassed to reveal what I usually eat: fruit, scrambled eggs, chocolate, and the occasional frozen Amy's meal. Pictures of salads cast me in a better light, right?

The second week goes better. I begin experimenting with incorporating other foods. I become adept at sandwiches and make one that I used to eat at a coffee shop during graduate school: hummus, sprouts, carrots, and apples on a baguette. Lunch in general includes more variety: I sometimes have peanut butter and jelly, and I include a few salads. I add a tortilla wrap to my longtime eggs, avocado, and salsa combo. I try new foods for breakfast. I prepare waffles with almond butter and bananas layered on top, and I begin making açai bowls. But dinners remain a challenge. I have pasta with chicken a few times. I substitute more frozen meals for the chocolate that has become my mainstay. But little changes.

Counseling plods along for a few months. I struggle to challenge my rigid thoughts about my body. I'm only an assistant professor in the humanities, and Dalit's fees are steep. I end counseling at the end of March 2019, and I stop taking photos of my food within the same week.

A year goes by. During the COVID-19 lockdown, food restriction helps me contain my anxiety. While others complain about weight gain, I become self-conscious about my eating habits and my gradual weight loss. Like everyone around me, I'm anguished, but I don't eat for comfort. I never have. Ever since I became self-conscious about food and weight around puberty, I've always restricted my food intake when I'm stressed. Whether it's a break-up or pressure at work, my appetite disappears when I'm burdened with anxiety or sadness.

One night, I have a Zoom dinner with my friend Elizabeth. Carrot soup is the choice that evening. I haven't followed any recipe. Boiled carrots and vegetable stock blended. I complain to her that it's both watery and lumpy at the same time. She recommends making it heartier with potatoes. I'm still hungry by the end of the meal. But I don't care enough to make any changes in my cooking. My fear of weight gain continues to haunt me. It makes little sense as I see my body wither away over the weeks. Still, I have a hard time modifying a recipe to make it more filling.

WHEN I FIRST BEGAN restricting my food intake as a teenager, I did not set out to be ill, and I never would have imagined being unable to care for myself or a loved one, like my dog. Instead, what I experienced was a decades-long slide from restriction to a diagnosable eating disorder. As I noted in chapter 1, many factors beyond weight-loss dieting predict disordered eating. Nevertheless, as psychologists have observed, dieting is the most common predictor of anorexia and bulimia. Whether it takes a few months or several decades, the slide I experienced is not uncommon.

In this chapter, I'll chart the landscape of disordered eating during the COVID-19 pandemic, a period that saw a noticeable rise in restrictive eating disorders, which calls for explanation. Did the fear of "pandemic pounds" drive this rise? Or was it the tendency to focus on one's appearance that new levels of videoconferencing brought? Or did the decline in access to mental health care in the early months of the pandemic lay the ground for this surge? I believe that these are all contributing factors. Yet there might also be a deeper reason behind the trend: For some individuals, disordered eating served as a coping mechanism during a moment of significant stress. If you or someone you know eats more or less in times of stress, you might recognize this pattern, whether or not it leads to a full-fledged disorder. So as we explore these hypotheses, I'll also break down an important philosophical concept: the notion of the *sublime*.

Mastering Fear, Mastering Hunger

To shed light on these pandemic-era changes, it's helpful to turn to a distinction made in philosophy between the beautiful and the sublime, which can be traced as far back as the ancient philosopher Aristotle.

It became prominent, however, in the eighteenth century. Immanuel Kant's *Critique of Judgment* develops one of the most common explanations of this distinction. Kant uses the language of *beauty* to characterize aesthetic experiences that afford a "positive pleasure." For instance, beholding a flower—appreciating its color and symmetry—might provide an experience of the beautiful. He introduces the category of the *sublime* to describe experiences linked to awe and wonder. For him, seemingly infinite objects can provoke this sense; when we look up at a starry sky and try to grapple with its vastness, we may enjoy a feeling of the sublime. Things that have the potential for destruction can also generate such an experience: for example, a storm or an erupting volcano.[1] Both cases—the infinite and the potentially destructive—give us a "negative pleasure." That is, unlike the beautiful, the pleasure of the sublime is tainted with fear.[2]

In "Sublime Hunger: A Consideration of Eating Disorders Beyond Beauty," the feminist thinker Sheila Lintott draws on this distinction. She explains that popular discourse around anorexia and bulimia doesn't go far enough when it conceives of beauty culture as the main driver of these disorders. The picture is more complicated. For some people, weight-loss dieting can become extreme and set the stage for an eating disorder. As Lintott puts it, while beauty "may start many women on the path to developing an eating disorder," appealing to the category of beauty is insufficient to understand what "keeps many on that path."[3] Instead, if we are to understand the motivations behind anorexia and bulimia, we need to consider the role of the sublime.

The sublime compels us to master our desire to run away in fear before a destructive object. Lintott argues that the mastery of hunger inherent in eating disorders gives women an experience of this feeling that they might not otherwise have access to. Her account emphasizes the feeling of self-worth that anorectics and bulimics derive from overcoming their hunger. "The dieter might truly wish her appetite to vanish, whereas the anorectic or bulimic depends on her hunger for her identity."[4] Specifically, anorectics and bulimics seek a sense of spirituality by overcoming their hunger, just what a mountaineer might chase by conquering a difficult ascent. Mastering hunger—not the appearance of thinness—eventually becomes part of one's identity in anorexia and bulimia.

Philosophers like Kant have claimed that both the beautiful and the sublime offer a sense of *pleasure*. His concept of the beautiful helps capture the pleasure we derive from adorning our bodies and the delight that comes with experimenting with new fashions or makeup styles. That is what philosophers have in mind when they refer to a "positive" pleasure from beauty. On the flip side, though, Lintott finds Kant's idea of "negative pleasure" relevant to the psychology of anorexia and bulimia. According to her analysis, there is something both satisfying and painful in conquering hunger. Marya Hornbacher's memoir of anorexia and bulimia, *Wasted*, makes vivid Kant's account. She uses the language of fear to elucidate her experience: "Some fear death, some seek it, but it is in our nature to wonder at the limits of human life, at least. When you are sick like this, you begin to wonder too much. Death is at your shoulder, death is your shadow, your scent, your waking and dreaming companion."[5] She adds that in pondering the possibility of her death, she also felt a sense of "longing."[6] Her description of being haunted by death speaks to the combination of fear and desire that her illness caused—an echo of the Kantian idea of pleasure being tainted with fear.

It's worth emphasizing that Lintott's theory focuses on women. She explains that women have been afforded fewer opportunities to confront the sublime in its traditional forms (for example, through extreme physical activities or exploration).[7] That's why they may turn to disordered eating behaviors to experience a feeling of control. Of course, there may be other factors in explaining the gender gap she had in mind when she discussed these disorders in 2003. But some people may recognize their experiences in her idea of defeating "an enemy"—namely, one's hunger.

How does this relate to the COVID-19 pandemic? Following Lintott's connection of disordered eating and the sublime, let's ask whether the fears brought on by the pandemic motivated some people to channel their energies into vanquishing their hunger. If mastering the pandemic was beyond our individual possibilities, controlling our hunger could still contribute to a form of agency and a sense of self-mastery.

Mastering Hunger, Mastering the Pandemic

Besides the threat of severe illness and death, the pandemic came with many disruptions to ordinary life. Reports of an increase in eating disorders at the time reveal how deeply these disruptions affected us. Although anecdotal evidence of the rising prevalence of eating disorders is plentiful, I take my cues from a retrospective analysis of studies of eating disorders during this period. Based on this analysis, the editorial board of the *International Journal of Eating Disorders* states: "The studies paint a worrisome, albeit somewhat mixed picture of the impact of the pandemic on eating symptomatology, as experienced by patients or individuals who self-report an eating disorder. Overall, if not always a majority, then still a considerable subset of participants reported a deterioration of their eating disorder symptoms."[8]

So a host of informal reports and empirical studies document an uptick in disordered eating. But why did we see this change? Put simply, our ongoing fixation on the beauty ideal of slenderness may not alone have caused the rise in the prevalence of eating disorders. Something deeper was going on.

The pandemic, at least during the lockdown phase, deprived many of us of our sense of agency. Unless we were on the front lines or working in medical research, those who lived in privileged circumstances, especially people who were alone, sought some mechanism to cope with this global threat. Some of us turned to creative hobbies—baking, knitting, art. And some of us developed problematic habits. Consider the rise in alcohol consumption. According to a 2023 NIH retrospective, "Alcohol sales jumped by nearly 3%, the largest increase in more than 50 years. Multiple small studies suggest that during the pandemic, about 25% of people drank more than usual, often to cope with stress."[9]

So just as people familiarly turn to alcohol to numb stress, some of us with a predisposition for disordered eating naturally turned to dieting to numb the anxiety brought by the pandemic. That's why the rise in eating disorders may be partially attributed to living in an overpowering situation, one that we tried to manage using food. And while I have focused on restrictive eating in this book, I should mention that data suggest that binge eating also worsened during the early days of the pandemic. "Recent evidence suggested that binge episodes increased with the outbreak of the pandemic," notes a 2024 study, "reaching peaks of 14% in young adults during the first lockdown period. . . . The increase in emotion-driven eating during the pandemic has been generally explained as a response to stressful experiences and emotional impairments associated with the health emergency."[10] Therefore, it's reasonable to expect that the adverse life events caused by the pandemic, with their negative emotional consequences, may have triggered binge eating in vulnerable individuals, resembling the negative effects of other traumatic experiences. Emma Specter's memoir *More, Please* chronicles this shift.[11] Specter had suffered from a binge eating disorder for years, but the pandemic led to increased bingeing and pushed her to confront her eating issues head-on. After this turning point, she persisted in counseling, which gave her the resources to make progress with challenging her disordered habits.

One hypothesis for the increase in disordered eating behaviors would be the fear of "pandemic pounds." People worried about the "COVID 15," an allusion to the "freshman 15" trope about weight gain in the first year of college. During lockdown many of us had less access to physical exercise, which may have led to weight gain. That said, one report indicates that "compared with the pre-pandemic weight trend, there was a small increase (0.1 kg) in weight in the first year of the pandemic."[12] The data is complicated by the fact that some people lost weight during the pandemic, which could have been due to stress or healthier food choices.[13] Altogether the statistics point to a mixed picture, with weight changes going in both directions. Still, we may wonder about the origin of some of these changes: Did popular (fat-phobic) discourse about weight gain lead to the spike in disordered eating behaviors based on food restriction?

A second hypothesis is that the increase in videoconferencing incentivized a focus on the body's appearance. This issue would naturally have affected those taking online classes or working in professions dependent on face-to-face meetings. Not only did we look at others while on Zoom or other platforms, but we were faced with images of ourselves on camera. According to a 2023 paper on a study in Australia, videoconferencing may not have been a driving factor in body dissatisfaction or restrictive eating during the pandemic. "Consistent with expectations, state-based videoconferencing use was associated with an increase in state-level urges to engage in exercise. However, contrary to predictions, state-based videoconferencing use was linked to a decrease in state-level BD (body dissatisfaction) at the next assessment point and failed to predict negative mood and urges to engage in restrictive eating or overeating/purging at the state level," the researchers said.[14] Of course, studies like this have their limits, but what is interesting for our purposes is that videoconferencing alone did not predict restrictive and binge-purge eating. If these findings hold up, then they may show that the turn to Zoom and other platforms did not straightforwardly drive the increase in disordered eating. If food restriction and other disordered eating patterns did increase, what other factors could explain it?

A third possible factor behind pandemic eating disorder trends was the change in access to mental health care. The switch from in-person care to telehealth for those already in treatment may have disrupted efforts to recover from disordered eating. A 2021 study of this shift noted that there was some correlation between the changes in care and worsening eating disorder symptoms, but that the patient's perception of the quality of their care (either positive or negative) predicted differences in symptoms.[15] This data may help us understand why individuals experiencing eating disorders continued to face challenges or relapsed during the pandemic, consistent with the ways I myself struggled. Another consideration worth envisioning is that people who were not yet in counseling but wanted help were having greater difficulty obtaining healthcare.

One study that may help us home in on this topic looked at "pandemic-related changes in social media use, body satisfaction, and perceived loss of control."[16] The researchers found that the pandemic negatively affected both healthy teenage girls and those suffering from anorexia, but girls with an eating disorder were more likely to feel a loss of personal control and turn to food restriction to cope with it.[17] This connection fits with earlier frameworks about the motivations behind anorexia and speaks directly to Lintott's appeal to the sublime to explain the origin of some disordered eating patterns: Restrictive eating may have been one way of trying to gain a sense of mastery during the pandemic.

Another key aspect of this study was the finding that alexithymia—difficulty identifying and describing one's own emotions—was also correlated with restrictive eating behavior.[18] This condition, also known as emotional blindness, can appear alongside autism spectrum disorders, depression, post-traumatic stress, and other conditions, as well as brain injuries.[19] Could the presence of alexithymia explain why, in the absence of a clear vocabulary for their emotions, people predisposed to disordered eating turned to restriction during the pandemic? Did disordered eating help them cope with a feeling that they could not *name*? These questions again raise the possibility that the philosophical category of the sublime, with its connotation of awe and fear, is pertinent.

The thrust of my argument is that, regardless of access to healthcare, some people may have experienced negative mental health because of the pandemic and turned to disordered eating as a coping mechanism. A host of factors likely caused the surge in eating disorder symptomatology, and psychologists are still working to assess their relevance. Considering these possible explanations and their limitations, it's still worth entertaining the idea that the pandemic was a unique stressor, one whose vastness overwhelmed many. To return to Lintott, while the thinness-beauty equation may have predisposed some of us to excessive dieting, it's the power of the pandemic, the sublime contained within it, that heightened disordered eating.

Beyond the Pandemic: Disordered Eating in Periods of Global Stress

In chapter 5, we examined the shortcomings of the body positivity movement that flourished in the 2010s, and noted how the popularization of GLP-1s starting in 2022 further damaged the movement's influence. I also sketched a path forward for body positivity, one where we consider other aspects of the body besides its appearance when seeking to heal from body dissatisfaction, and one where we recognize that some persons are more vulnerable than others because of weight stigma and related harms.

That discussion overlaps with the points I've made in this chapter. I've suggested that the unexpected and unusual stress of the pandemic exacerbated disordered eating, both binge eating and restrictive eating. And an interesting aspect of the human condition in this disorder, at least for restrictive eating, is the attempt to master our fear of the sublime by mastering our hunger. Now let's look ahead. What would a society look like where eating behaviors did not become a coping mechanism? For one, thinness would have less of a hold on us as a beauty ideal. We would be more attuned to our bodies through physical practices, especially those that lend us strength as subjects *in* our bodies, rather than those that merely motivate us to look *at* our bodies. Besides this, to honor the idea that some are more vulnerable than others, we would also need to overcome the social isolation that's conducive to harmful ways of dealing with stressors. We must ask: How can we weaken the connection between denying oneself food and self-transcendence? And how can we strengthen the link between nourishing oneself and self-care? The next chapter will consider these questions.

My reckoning with disordered eating comes within a year of the start of the pandemic. On the night when food restriction prevents me from taking my dog on her usual walk, I know I must return to counseling. The day after, I call the practice where I used to see my counselor, Dalit. I will meet with her on September 29, 2020. My first time seeing her in over a year.

Will I mention the moment when my world collapsed? That's the reason I'm going back to counseling. But can I summon the courage to share the moment when I realized I could no longer live like this anymore?

Will I reveal my shameful conduct—my drunkenness, my inability to care for Carol? I ruminate with the cursor hovering above the Zoom login link she has sent me. As my laptop clock ticks to 2 p.m., I join the meeting.

There she is: Dalit. She looks the same. The same delicate smile as during our first round of counseling. The same dark hair pulled tightly back. But I can no longer see any colorful outfit. I miss seeing people's outfits. I miss reading others' body language. I miss relaxing into the plush chair at her practice. Instead, I sit upright in bed. Thus begins my second round of eating disorder counseling.

Interlude

A Test Subject

Ten days after resuming eating disorder counseling, I find myself at my annual physical. It's a coincidence that the appointment is scheduled so close to the beginning of my therapy "take #2." Since Dalit is conducting counseling by Zoom, there is no other way to record my weight but at the doctor's office. During my first round of counseling, she would weigh me in her office. Dalit never talks of my buying myself a scale. Down my weight would go, and down with it would go any chance at recovery.

I guess that I must weigh less than 130 pounds. My ribs stick out, and the recent restricting that led to the moment when I felt my world collapse hint at that. Since the pandemic, I've been struggling with my eating again, and a few months into a whirlwind romance, a person I've been dating breaks things off. I fell for her fast, so fast that when she announced on the phone one night that she didn't "feel any chemistry," I understood for the first time the significance of the phrase "being punched in the gut." I did not eat for a day. Two months into this pain and confusion, I still can't shake my sadness over the end of our romance. Now I suspect that I've hit the number that once was my holy grail: 125.

A nurse calls my name. I jump up, brace my handbag against my side, and walk up to her. She scans my forehead to read my temperature. All clear. I enter the examination room, where she motions me to place my bag down and hop on the scale.

My heart beats so wildly that I dread having my pulse and blood pressure measured next. What will the nurse think? She'll conclude that I'm deathly ill, or I'll have to explain how much I dread being weighed. Perhaps I can avoid these outcomes by not looking at the scale.

I step onto the machine and fix my eyes on the wall ahead. Despite my obsession with thinness, no matter how low the number, I hate, just hate, being weighed. I've trained myself not to look down.

The light on the scale flashes, and I hear the nurse scribble something on a notepad. I've been weighed.

I step off and steady myself onto the examination table. The nurse hooks me up to the blood pressure machine, takes my pulse, and straps a tiny oxygen meter to one of my fingers. She reads my vitals and makes no comment. I wonder if avoiding seeing the number on the scale has helped steady my racing heart.

There's now a grave problem, though. By not looking at the number, I've failed to gather the information that's crucial for Dalit at the beginning of this new round of eating disorder counseling. The only way I'm going to get it is by asking the nurse. But I have no time to interject as she starts asking me customary questions about my smoking, drinking, coffee consumption habits, etc. My answers blur into one another. And my mind races even faster than my heartbeat pre-weigh-in. How will I get the information I need? I know from previous visits that she's nearing the end of her tedious questions. Finally, just as she exits the room for me to undress, I whisper, "How much did I weigh? I need to let my eating disorder counselor know." The nurse glances at a piece of paper. "125."

I've failed myself. That's the only thought that reverberates in the silence left by the nurse. I've failed myself. I've failed myself.

I take my time undressing. I let the number sink in. From having obsessively calculated my BMI over the years, I know that my weight makes my BMI just shy of 17. The BMI is bogus, I've read again and again, especially in progressive critiques of the healthcare system. Still, keeping that number in the underweight range had been a source of pride. But 17 is not just in the "underweight" bracket, it's starting to dip pretty low, bad low. How bad it is will depend on the assessment used. Roughly, I've slid from the "mild thinness" category to "moderate/severe thinness" one. From the benign to the harmful.

Fifteen minutes elapse before the doctor knocks on the door. "May I come in?"

In comes a man in his fifties with graying hair and deep creases in his cheeks. He's tall, slim, and stern-looking. He gives off a generic doctor gravitas. He strides in with a medical intern, whom he's allowing to do the intake. She's a twentysomething blonde girl, definitely younger than I am, and she's smiling. From my perspective, she seems eager to please him. It's a teaching hospital, and I've complied with these requests for years. He leaves the room.

My self-flagellating thoughts distract me so much that I don't notice her questions until she reaches my family history. Weakened, I can only mumble the answers she needs. She takes notes on a clipboard with a paper full of tables whose words I cannot decipher from my angle. "Do you have any medical conditions in your family?" "My mother has high blood pressure, and my father has no diseases I know of." "And your grandparents?" "They're all dead." "What were their causes of death?" She's about to scribble these down, too, in one of the Excel-like boxes. Mamie's cause of death was complications of hemochromatosis. I don't remember if she says "how cool" or "how interesting." What is seared in me, though, is that she's smiling widely as she tells me how she learned about this genetic condition in her first year of med school and now gets to hear about it firsthand! How dare you look at me with that gleeful look? I'm telling you how my grandmother died. I don't have the nerve to tell her how badly she's messed up.

She spins around like a marionette, head high, with her clipboard under her arm—exit Perfect Resident. I'm pained and want nothing to do with her.

A few minutes go by. I'm already shaking from the whole ordeal: I'm disappointed with myself for letting my eating problems get this bad and I'm annoyed by the med school student. I anchor myself with my hands, knotted around the chair's frame: I cannot betray any emotion to the doctor, or I'd let on how bad things have gotten. I'm too stoic for that. Plus, he doesn't seem like the type to talk about emotions.

Enter the Perfect Resident, this time with Unemotional Doctor behind her. I'm seated. She looks down at me while he stands ready, stage left.

She glances down at her clipboard, looks directly at him, and chirps: "The patient is a thirty-four-year-old woman with anorexia and a history of depression . . ."

Anorexia. My mind fixates on the word and I lose the rest of what she says.

For her, I'm a neat test subject: someone who needs to be sized up efficiently for what is "wrong." But for me, something decisive has happened. What happens occupies my thoughts more loudly than the review of my health data, my sadness about the recently ended romance, or the feeling of that I let myself down, down all the way to 125. What is louder than this in my mind is that I'm finally met with the term that no one has ever uttered to my face. Until that moment, I've used the vague terms "eating issues" and "body image problems." Others had echoed my language.

But here is the verdict. "Anorexia." That's the diagnosis.

PART 2

What Do We Do Now?

7

Eating, Cooking, and the Ethics of Self-Care

Caring for myself is not self-indulgence, it is self-preservation, and that is an act of political warfare.

—AUDRE LORDE, *A Burst of Light*

In February 2021, several months after I resume eating disorder counseling with my therapist, Dalit, I begin virtual cooking lessons with my mother. I've spent the intervening time attempting to cook more wholesome meals and trying to prepare dinners, the meal I had most often skipped. I begin with my mother's recipe for pasta Bolognese. Every Saturday evening, I cook the dish and am gaining a sense of mastery from perfecting it. In the new year, however, I start to grow bored with my weekly feast. I don't remember how I come up with the idea of having my mother teach me new recipes. Is it my own invention? Or a suggestion by my therapist? Regardless, I float it by my mother one day: Since we cannot see each other as often as we did before the pandemic, I want her to teach me how to cook virtually.

Our first recipe is "Chinese chicken." This is a vague label she has come up for two dishes: one version with chicken, the other with pork. Both consist of meat cooked in a spicy sauce along with bell peppers and pineapples, and served with white rice.

My mother texts me the list of ingredients, and I lay them out: chicken breasts, a can of pineapple chunks, flour, white wine, soy sauce, sunflower seed oil, white wine vinegar, fresh ginger, a large green pepper, a large tomato, an onion, crushed chili peppers, powdered sugar, salt, and rice. I live in a studio apartment, and the spread takes up most of my kitchen's counterspace. As would become my custom, I forget an important element of the "mise en place": the ingredients are all there, but I've failed to measure them. I'll have to do it as we go along. This first snafu doesn't dampen my excitement: I'm starting to like the idea of cooking and look forward to my mother's companionship.

I prop my phone against my paper towel rack and pour myself a glass of wine, something my mother does while cooking. My phone rings at six o'clock sharp. She begins by instructing me to cut the chicken into small pieces. Luckily, I have meat scissors, one of the few cooking utensils I acquired before learning how to cook. Then we sprinkle the pieces with flour and sauté them in white wine and soy sauce for two minutes. Meanwhile, I prepare the ginger, green pepper, and onion; once they're minced, they're cooked together for three minutes. I find cleaning tomatoes of their seeds tedious, but my mother insists that it needs to be done thoroughly. In they go, seedless and diced, along with powdered sugar, flour, crushed chili peppers, soy sauce, vinegar, and the juice from the can of pineapple chunks. I cook them for ten minutes as we catch up about work. I realize that I need to start boiling the water for rice. As I eye the timer on the rice, I continue to stir the vegetables before adding the pineapples. The timer on my phone rings. The rice has caught up with the rest of the meal. I thank my mother for the cooking lesson, hang up the phone, and promise to tell her how I like it.

The dish tastes much like the one she has prepared since my childhood. I remember the time when she used such spicy peppers that our dogs—Sparky and Cinnamon—started choking on the fumes. She had to rush out of the apartment with them in tow, and I found them waiting outside the front door when I returned from a music lesson. My version is tamer: spicy but not overpoweringly so, sweet, and a bit tangy. Despite the kitchen's disarray, I feel a sense of peace. I'm enjoying my food without worrying about its calorie content. Later, as that lesson grows into years of weekly sessions, I cherish the nourishment—physical and spiritual—the meals bring with them.

YOU'VE NOW FOLLOWED my analysis of the forces of modern society that shape our perspectives on beauty, nourishment, and health. And you've followed my own personal journey of responding and reacting to these forces, beginning with my innocent indulgence in blueberry tarts as a young girl, then through my struggle to manage the new messaging about beauty and diet that is part of "becoming" a woman, and finally to the moment when I was confronted with a diagnosis of anorexia that could no longer be ignored.

Now the questions are these: When we reach this point, how do we pick ourselves back up? What ideas and strategies return the power we have unwittingly given away? And how can we not merely survive but thrive in the face of our mistakes—emerging stronger, wiser, and more capable of passing on our wisdom to others?

The rest of this book is my answer to these questions. And it all begins with a thought—the essential role of developing *practices* to bring any of my recommendations into your life as richly as possible. My idea is this: In response to social forces that do not care for us, we need to care for ourselves. In response to social forces that want us to be weak and dependent, we need to rise up and liberate ourselves. In response to social forces that starve us, we need to nourish ourselves. And we need to do this not as an easily forgotten platitude, but in a way that animates our lives. We begin this journey of wisdom and empowerment at what might seem like an unlikely place: cooking lessons. Yes, food not as an act of denial or brush with death, but as a way to be present in the world, to touch life and earth, and to come into true community.

The practices in this part of the book stem from a simple question: *What role does self-care play in eating disorder recovery and resistance to diet culture?* As we investigate this topic, we'll take an overview of the ideal of self-care before moving on to the idea that intuitive eating—a practice I'll soon define—can be a form of self-care. The insights we'll gain also apply to cultivating "intuitive movement"—that is, forms of movement that are not driven by appearance concerns and that honor our bodily abilities (which we'll cover in chapter 8).

Where Did the Self-Care Ideal Come From?

The education expert Christopher Ziguras writes that "'self-care' refers to the active process of recovering, maintaining and improving one's health."[1] Some self-care practices are physical maintenance—cleaning our teeth, getting rest, avoiding injuries. In healthcare fields, self-care typically refers to the practices that an individual can engage in to restore their health (e.g., taking medication). But when we think of self-care, we often have more in mind than taking meds or flossing. It has a broader significance and includes "those everyday practices in which people engage to maintain or improve their own health."[2] As Ziguras phrases it, self-care practices "are not so much techniques of the body as 'techniques of the self' aimed at sustaining mental health by managing one's self-identity, self-perception, feelings, and relationships."[3] Most practices spotlighted on social media or in self-help books speak only to the "health-enhancing" strand of self-care.

To dig deeper into this powerful idea, let's consider its origins. When I began my second round of eating disorder counseling, I was aware of the idea of "care of the soul" from my education in philosophy. In the *Apology*, Plato depicts the trial of his teacher, Socrates, who had been charged with corrupting the youth of Athens and not worshipping the gods of the city, among other things. During the trial, Socrates was found guilty. In his response to this verdict, he reflected on the conversations that had led to these accusations: "I spend my whole life in going about and persuading you all to give your first and greatest care to the well-being of your souls, and not till you have done that to think of your bodies or your wealth."[4] I interpreted him as saying that caring for one's soul meant attending to the details of daily life that support one's mental health. For him, engaging in philosophical dialogue is one way to care for oneself, as are intellectual pursuits and regulating our desires. Personal appearance and riches don't determine the content of happiness—the quality of our relationships and our search for wisdom do. Despite my familiarity with this text and many other dialogues by Plato featuring Socrates, I'd never appreciated the connection between his ideas and my own life. I'd grown tired of seeing bubble bath and spa day photos under #selfcare on Instagram, and these images seemed superficial compared to his advice. Sure, a spa day could help calm my nerves after a stressful workweek. But what did this have to do with seeking wisdom?

In another dialogue featuring Socrates, the *Phaedo*, Plato elaborates that the soul of the philosopher is one not tainted by easy indulgence in the body's appetites, such as lust and hunger, but rather one who goes beyond that in search of a grander, intellectual way of being. When we indulge in our intellect, we seek to grasp the essences of those things we encounter in our life. But such a search is difficult. The essence of a triangle (i.e., a three-sided planar figure) may be easy to get, but that of beauty or goodness is harder to understand. So for Plato and Socrates, we care for ourselves by avoiding *mindless* indulgence of our appetites, and instead carefully studying the essences of the things we encounter. Because of my own struggles, I don't share the same worries about the body and its appetites. Still, there's tremendous value in the idea that *mindful* life choices matter to caring for oneself. For me, learning to take pleasure in food and to cook were—perhaps paradoxically—the ways I came to embody their vision of self-care.

After Plato's death, the tradition of caring for oneself branched out from Athens to the rest of the ancient Western world. Take the philosopher Epicurus, who lived over a century later. He claimed that moderating certain forms of enjoyment laid the groundwork for a good life. Contrary to our current conception of self-care, where more lavish approaches, such as luxurious wellness retreats, seem to be the norm, being an Epicurean was about living in a way that is not bored by but finds delight and insight in simple pleasures. As the contemporary commentator Emily Austin has noted, Epicurus's background ideas about the nature of the universe—it consists of atoms and void—are more compatible with modern science than those of other thinkers in Antiquity.[5] His claims about pleasure still feel applicable, too. Epicurus taught that chasing ever grander pleasures (e.g., buying the latest trendy accessory that you'll replace with an even trendier and more expensive one next month) would backfire in the long run.[6] Such a chase creates never-ending expectations as we grow tired of each luxury after another. It's better to keep things simple and satisfy our physical and mental needs. Although I'd taught Epicurus for many years, including during those when I suffered from disordered eating, I'd never realized how relevant his ideas were to my condition. I imagine he would have found my desire to appear thin and conform to punitive beauty standards to be a groundless or vain pursuit.

The ancients also described practices that contributed to self-transformation at an intellectual level. One Stoic practice is that of "negative visualization," which requires imagining the negative events that may happen to you so that you're better prepared for them. For example, in his *Meditations*, the Roman emperor Marcus Aurelius asserts, "Begin the morning by saying to thyself, I shall meet with the busybody, the ungrateful, arrogant, deceitful, envious, unsocial. All these things happen to them by reason of their ignorance of what is good and evil."[7] As an application of this idea, for a person who is underweight and captivated by the beauty industry, imagine yourself a few pounds heavier, but having spent the time on self-development, also a few ticks smarter, more social, and happier.

Like other ancient values, such as taking joy in simple pleasures, self-care made a "comeback" in the modern West after being eclipsed by Christian ethical principles for centuries. As the writer Jordan Kisner notes, "Historically, in America, full citizenship has rested on an idea of the capacity for self-care."[8] For example, a lack of self-care was used to justify slavery. In the nineteenth century, the physician Samuel A. Cartwright spoke of a "debasement of mind, which has rendered the people of Africa unable to take care of themselves."[9] Similarly, a few decades later, immigrants from Southern and Eastern Europe were "deemed 'unfit citizens' because they lacked the 'ideas and attitudes which befit men to take up . . . the problem of self-care and self-governance.'"[10] This line of reasoning made the capacity for self-care a qualification for citizenship and served to support anti-democratic positions, despite the optimistic associations with the idea I've provided so far.

During the first half of the twentieth century, the notion of self-care faded away. Yet Kisner mentions that "after decades of disuse, the term [self-care] was repopularized in the seventies and eighties by people of color and queer communities—this time as a gesture of defiance."[11] Here, he has in mind the feminist writer Audre Lorde, whose powerful quote opened this chapter: "Caring for myself is not self-indulgence, it is self-preservation and that is an act of political warfare."[12] Lorde penned these words in her 1988 book *A Burst of Light*, which detailed her experience with treatments for breast cancer. She sought several medical opinions about her condition and traveled to pursue alternative medicine treatments. On a superficial reading, you could say that she was just trying to heal from her illness. Why make her actions into a statement of political protest? I think that her position as a member of several oppressed groups challenged the presumption that Black lives like hers were expendable. For Lorde, marginalized members of society, alternately neglected or vilified, often felt themselves unworthy of care. But when they chose to care for themselves, their actions became instances of political resistance.

In recent years, self-care has branched into two ideals. On the one hand, some communities have continued Lorde's legacy. For instance, Kisner cites the case of a Black trans man, Devin-Norelle, who, after the killings of Philando Castile and Alton Sterling, "posted a mostly naked self-portrait with the comment 'Healing is self-care is self-love, self-indulgence, and self-preservation, because sometimes we need to be reminded that #BlackIsBeautiful.'"[13] For people like Devin-Norelle, self-care serves as a form of self-protection against continued social injustices. On the other hand, self-care has also become increasingly coopted and commodified. On social media, under #selfcare, proliferate photos of wellness treatments embraced by people living in privileged circumstances. One concern about this trend is that it feels like a balm for those who are overburdened by fast-paced corporate careers, rather than a stance of resistance to the economic situations driving burnout. Indeed, in *Real Self-Care*, Pooja Lakshmin indicates that instead of seeking flashy displays of self-care, we need to change the very situations, for example, hostile work environments, that compel us to go to expensive yoga classes or buy fancy bubble bath sets.[14] More than that, we need to place less of a burden on individuals experiencing burnout to advocate for improved situations—we must *collectively* seek ways to create better working conditions. Something similar could be said of less-conspicuous displays of self-care: Consider the case of someone who's chastised for buying a cup of coffee instead of making it at home when they're struggling to pay bills. Even here, we need to think more broadly about remedies rather than judging individual choices. The long-term solution will be to improve our economy in equitable ways so that people don't find themselves in these financial difficulties. We'll need to craft and enact changes that bring about social justice, rather than reaching for shortcuts.

The fact that self-care has branched into two such different ideals should remind us that all good ideas can be coopted and interpreted in ways that no longer preserve their original intent. So it's important for us to be vigilant about the idea of self-care, and careful in making connections. While a bubble bath could count as a nice thing to do for oneself, true self-care requires a much more comprehensive practice—one that is aware of the numerous social forces that seem to try to prevent us from caring for ourselves deeply. This is a good moment for us to slow down and consider one of the common criticisms of the self-care ideal, namely that it breeds narcissism.

Is Self-Care Narcissistic?

Let's begin with a description by Christopher Ziguras of why people grew interested in self-care in the United States. The 1970s saw a growing concern about traditional Western medical practices; alongside grew an interest in alternative treatments based on non-Western healing traditions. At the same time, people wanted to take greater ownership of their well-being. Self-help books began to crop up, as did new diets (e.g., juicing) or therapies (e.g., "scream therapy"). These shifts coalesced into the ideal of caring for oneself, and in some circles, it was conceived of as a political practice. Critics of self-care found this "inward shift" narcissistic.[15] They argued that self-care enthusiasts were focused on themselves as opposed to their responsibilities as family members or citizens. Among them, Christopher Lasch claimed that therapeutic systems cut people off from others and created a form of social withdrawal.[16] These systems discouraged "investment in love and friendship" and "excessive dependence on others," thereby exacerbating "the very conditions that created the crisis of personal relations in the first place."[17] Here, he has in mind problems like loneliness and feelings of meaninglessness. I think this is too superficial a reading of the situation. It misses the point that self-care is not *necessarily* narcissistic, since we can also learn to care for others by first engaging in self-care.

Myisha Cherry, a contemporary philosopher and an expert on Audre Lorde, argues that self-care and what she calls "solidarity care" can be in conversation with one another. In "Solidarity Care: How to Take Care of Each Other in Times of Struggle," she outlines the burdens that oppression places on people. First, these burdens can be "existential," like twentieth-century African American sociologist W. E. B. Du Bois's idea of double consciousness—the pain of seeing yourself through the eyes of the privileged, the feeling of "being a problem" in society.[18] Second, oppression can take a psychological toll on us. As an illustration, Cherry mentions the race-based traumatic stresses that Black Americans experience, which can lay the ground for severe conditions like psychosis.[19]

Cherry responds that we need collective care to shoulder these burdens. Simply focusing on gaining greater freedoms will not undo oppression; we also need to extend care to one another. Furthermore, she says, self-care depends on solidarity care: "Self-care is never done independently. Someone has to watch the kids as you meditate. Someone teaches the yoga class that relaxes you. Someone gifts you with the book that is changing your life. A therapist or friend listens to your story," she notes.[20]

My experience illustrates Cherry's argument: Thanks to my counselor, I recognized the value of learning how to cook, and thanks to my mother, I acquired that skill, which helped me care for myself. Later, once I grew confident enough to share my own baking, I cared for others. At the beginning of her article, Cherry quotes Lorde: "Without community there is no liberation, only the most vulnerable and temporary armistice between an individual and her oppression."[21] I also see the truth in these words. For years, I'd tried to reform my eating habits and resist rigid standards of beauty on my own. Yet none of my efforts had met with any lasting success. Rather, the care I received from my counselor, the support of my closest friends, and the lessons I received from my mother helped me make lasting peace with my food. Caring for oneself depends on others, and caring for others depends on caring for oneself. This connection, as obvious as it may seem, is easily forgotten.

Eating Disorder Recovery as Self-Care

Christopher Ziguras distinguishes between self-care conceived as restoring one's health and self-care as a practice akin to personal development. Let's draw on this distinction to explore the idea of eating-disorder recovery as self-care. Recovery from an eating disorder seems to squarely fit under the "health restoration" rubric. But for some people, including myself, recovery has a broader significance that mirrors the "personal development" part of his definition.

During the years I spent in counseling, I grew to develop intuitive eating habits. *Intuitive eating* refers to ways of nourishing oneself through food choices, honoring physical and emotional needs. In my experience, this meant eating when I was hungry and avoiding shortcuts like drinking water at the beginning of a meal to feel satiated more quickly.

Unlike in weight-loss dieting, appearance concerns don't shape intuitive eating choices. According to the Harvard Medical School, "Intuitive eating rejects the rules and restrictions baked into a diet mentality."[22] This approach to nutrition avoids the "yo-yo weight loss and gain" so often caused by dieting.[23] As a teenager, when I was operating under the norms of diet culture, I stuck to my pain au chocolat for lunch, regardless of how hungry I was. Thanks to counseling, however, I learned to eat in a more flexible manner that mirrored how much hunger I felt. This practice helped me overcome the years of restrictive eating that had warped my relationship with my hunger and my body.

Intuitive eating often has an important role in the lives of people recovering from anorexia or bulimia. That said, it might not play such a role right away. Anorectics and bulimics may need to begin with nutritional rehabilitation and weight restoration,[24] or eating protocols and behavioral changes. Someone who is suffering acutely from anorexia or bulimia may not be able to engage in intuitive eating because they have skewed hunger signals (for instance, very reduced ones). Or they may be hospitalized and being fed intravenously. Yet with weight restoration, their eating disorder recovery may branch out into acquiring intuitive eating habits.[25]

During the two and a half years I was in counseling, I steadily gained the weight needed for my optimal health thanks to intuitive eating. Besides the physical changes, I felt a sense of accomplishment as my cooking repertoire expanded from eggs for lunch to all the dinners my mother taught me: pasta Bolognese, "Chinese chicken," Moroccan couscous, beef bourguignon, stuffed bell peppers, penne alla vodka, and so many more. This mastery differed from that which restriction afforded. Whereas controlling my food intake involved denying my body's needs, cooking involved creativity. I transitioned from a "negative pleasure" to a "positive pleasure," to draw on the contrast between the sublime and the beautiful. Restricting signified self-denial; creating new meals meant self-development. This difference echoes Ziguras's idea that self-care can encompass personally transformative practices. In addition, because I was learning from someone else, cooking ended the isolation caused by my disordered eating. Of course, not everyone will take joy from preparing meals, and not everyone will have the opportunity to find guidance from others. That's why I'll consider other avenues toward reclaiming a wholesome relationship to one's body in the remaining chapters of this book.

Although I've found intuitive eating to be healing, I should also stress that more structured approaches might work better for other people. For instance, in her memoir *A Physical Education*, Casey Johnston describes how lifting weights helped her ditch diet culture. The strenuous activities she engaged in led her to favor tracking metrics like macronutrients to inform her food choices.[26] Johnston worries that intuitive eating can favor unhealthy selections. Years of eating processed foods, paired with our genetic tendency to seek high-sugar or high-fat meals, may make people crave these types of foods. This is a common concern about intuitive eating, founded on the idea that many of us have been consuming foods detrimental to physical health for so many years that we cannot make healthy food choices by merely following our "intuition." I am sympathetic to this worry. Would following my intuition lead me to consume milk chocolate nonstop? Perhaps you have the same question about your favorite junk food. But like the other ideas we're considering, the fact that it can be misunderstood or misapplied doesn't discredit intuitive eating altogether. Instead, this worry should compel us to find a balanced approach, where we first reacquaint ourselves with feelings of *hunger* and *fullness* and then transition to incorporating foods that can bolster our physical health in the long term. For some people, after spending their life calculating calories, using metrics could create a new opportunity for disordered eating behaviors. Yet for others, like Johnston, these metrics might open the door for more wholesome ways of eating. As with all the practices I developed as part of my recovery, I want to describe them in a way that calls attention to their benefits while also accounting for how they can be misunderstood. And I want to make it clear that I'm not suggesting that they will work for everyone. Indeed, part of genuine recovery, I believe, is developing open-mindedness, which includes the realization that we all have our own path to health and flourishing.

Can We Think of Eating Disorder Recovery as Political?

As we've seen in previous chapters, social forces such as sexism and racism have helped enshrine thinness in women as a beauty standard. The thinness norm drives diet culture, which, in turn, fuels some instances of disordered eating. If we work our way backward, we might ask the following questions: Does healing from disordered eating count as a resistance to diet culture? And does resistance to diet culture count as an "act of political warfare," to borrow from Lorde?

To answer these questions, it's helpful to have a few test cases in mind. First, imagine someone who knows deep down that they're harming themselves through their disorder but may not be aware of the political transformations that led to the thinness standard. In that case, I would be wary of calling their efforts to heal themselves—let's say through intuitive eating—acts of political resistance. It would be like claiming to protest an injustice when you inadvertently got swept up in a rally while on the way to the grocery store!

Second, suppose that someone is conscious of the historical origins of diet culture but only gestures at intuitive eating (for example, on social media), all the while continuing to cut corners with food. This kind of "performative activism" wouldn't count as healing, since the person isn't practicing what they preached.

There is a variation on the first case worth considering. Envision a person who's not aware of the social significance of their eating habits, but nevertheless models gentler approaches to nutrition, such as intuitive eating, to others around them. In that case, you might say that they contribute to the larger cause of challenging diet culture, but in a less political way than someone who is explicitly aware of the harms of fatphobia and its roots in sexism and racism. These cases suggest that not all instances of healing from disordered eating are political in nature, but *some* subset might be. A healing person would need to be both politically informed and actively trying to shape their eating habits in opposition to diet culture. Or in a more derivative way, their actions might inspire others to resist this culture.

In 2022, after my foray into cooking for myself, I decide it's time to learn how to bake. My sister joins my mother one afternoon on WhatsApp video. They'll prepare banana bread together and teach me along the way. Well into the pandemic, I'm belatedly joining the baking crew.

My mother's recipe is simple: bananas, butter, sugar, flour, one egg, vanilla extract, salt, and baking soda. I've already taken the ingredients out and preheated the oven to 350 degrees. Within fifteen minutes, we've joked our way through the preparation of the dough and references to "lockdown baking."

Fifty minutes later, I take the bread out of the oven and test it with a toothpick to make sure it's cooked through. It is. I snap a picture of the loaf, brown on the edges but blonde in the center, and add the photo to my "Food Journal" album that I share with my counselor. Dalit will be proud that I'm finally giving baking a shot. After the loaf has cooled, I sample a piece. I bite into one on the end: The crust is hard, but not crunchy, the inside is soft, slightly moist. The taste of banana is subtle. As someone who has a sweet tooth, I wonder if I should put more sugar in next time. Later, I'll learn that most of my friends, family, and students enjoy the lightly sweetened flavor.

Banana bread turns out to be so easy to bake that I introduce a new ritual. Besides weekly virtual cooking lessons with my mother, I bake banana bread every Monday. A month or two into my new routine, I realize that my bread is perhaps decent enough to share with others. My first guinea pig is Elizabeth, who had so gently encouraged me to make a heartier soup when I was struggling with eating during lockdown. I bring her some bread one morning, and she has a taste. "Really good." I try to decipher her expression. It's friendly, but I can't shake my insecurity. Does she really enjoy it? Or is she humoring me? Before eating disorder counseling, I was so reluctant to cook and dismissive of food that I'd never have imagined baking anything, let alone sharing it. But her reassurance feels genuine. Elizabeth is a Kantian. I've never known her to lie.

From then on, I bring her two slices every Tuesday before work. As she continues to appear to enjoy them, I take a second leap: I bake bread for several teas in the Philosophy Department at my university. At the first one, the students and faculty seem to appreciate the bread, too. Do I have a knack for this? I switch things up to improve the "hygiene factor" for the next tea. Instead of baking a loaf, I prepare banana bread mini muffins: No one needs to touch anyone else's food.

Four years after my first banana bread, I've kept to my ritual. I bake a loaf every Monday. I bring some to Elizabeth on Tuesday. I share banana bread mini muffins at departmental events. Every few months, I send some as a gift for a widowed friend of my mother's. To use Dalit's words, baking has become my "love language."

My grandmother, Mamie Maude, first taught me how to bake and savor food. She modeled a healthy relationship to cooking and eating. But she died too early for me to draw on her lessons to resist diet culture. These lessons were unlearned, or perhaps I should say they lay dormant for twenty-five years. I took the first step toward caring for myself as an adult when I sought counseling for disordered eating. This first step speaks to the conception of self-care as recovery. I was working to "restore" my weight, as Dalit would put it. When my mother showed me how to cook, however, I entered a new stage in my recovery. I deepened my relationship with her and appreciated the subtleties of good cooking. Thanks to her, I could truly embody self-care.

When I took the leap into baking for others, I carried my grandmother's and mother's lessons forward. I grasped the connection between self-care and solidarity care described by Myisha Cherry. Caring for the self is something that I learned from others, but also something that I hope to share. For members of marginalized social groups, the value of self-care is not merely a matter of ethics. Rather, as Lorde so powerfully proclaimed, self-care can be a political statement. Eating and cooking helped me shake the grasp of the tyranny of thinness. These practices may not have the same significance for everyone. As we'll see in the next chapters, other activities can help people struggling with diet culture, too. But in my experience, to paraphrase Lorde's words about self-care, "Cooking for myself is not self-indulgence, it is self-preservation, and that is an act of political warfare."

8

Resisting the Allure of Self-Objectification

Part of being a subject, Beauvoir thought, is allowing yourself, and your say, to be the object of other people's judgment, rational or irrational: to risk being ridiculed or condemned or ignored or, worse, to find yourself convinced that the harsh judgments of others are true—or, maybe worst of all, to be confused about these judgments, to discover that, after all, you don't know who you are. Here is where we are especially tempted to try to subvert the risk posed by other people's objectifying gazes by preemptively objectifying ourselves. . . . To the extent we repress this fact . . . we deny ourselves a certain wherewithal to resist the allure of self-objectification.

—NANCY BAUER, "Simone de Beauvoir on the Allure of Self-Objectification"

"Are you ready?"

I nod, and my friend Jess lets go of the steel bar. I feel its full weight for the first time.

My biceps shake and my abs clench as I lower it toward my chest. I pause for a moment and then steadily push the bar back up. I lower it again, and I feel the muscles in my back lock this time. I push the bar up.

Then I lower it a third time and push it back up. I nod to Jess, who helps me set the bar down. My first three bench presses.

I'm almost twenty-eight. I've exercised most of my adult life. As a college student, I wanted to lose or maintain my weight: Every other minute on the treadmill compensated for a ten-calorie indiscretion. In my mid-twenties, at the beginning of graduate school, I convert some of the time I spend walking outdoors into calorie compensation. I know how many I can burn walking three miles per hour (or four). But when a foot injury, contracted while running, prevents me from engaging in compulsive walking, I head to Hemenway Gymnasium at Harvard. I've heard that weightlifting can boost your metabolism. For the first time since becoming a member of my school's gym, I walk down the stairs to the lower level. Jess, and later two other women friends, will join me in venturing into the uncharted terrain of Hemenway's weight room.

During my first weeks of lifting, I assume that the new exercise will compensate for food indiscretions. Yet in the months that follow, the goal of cultivating strength starts to override my mental calorie calculus. I go from pulling forty pounds to fifty, from two sets of kettlebell swings to three, from three bench presses to six. During that period, I stop focusing on my thigh gap or checking thinspo sites. When I used to log miles on the treadmill, I would feel the need to dominate my body, to beat the hell out of it to conform to the models' physiques I idealized. On the lower level of the gym, I learn to control my muscles so I can grow stronger.

At Hemenway, I avoid the mirrors. I strive to cultivate strength for the feeling I have during and after my workouts—not for a muscular appearance. I am trying not to replace my preoccupation with the thigh gap with a new obsession over my appearance.

I FIRST PENNED this vignette in 2016, during my final year of graduate school, after a brief reprieve from my fascination with thinspo. Finishing my dissertation and moving to Miami disrupted those weightlifting days. My fixation on my body returned, and as I've described, it led to a diagnosable eating disorder during the pandemic. Once I began healing from this disorder, in part through learning to cook, I began to appreciate my body again *for what it could do*. In this chapter, let's explore the power of movement in resisting self-objectification and reclaiming a wholesome relationship to oneself.

In chapter 2, we first met the philosophical distinction between the body-as-subject and the body-as-object. Body-as-subject means that our body allows us to act upon the world and to perceive it. Through physical movement, we relate to the objects and persons around us. Jumping to catch a ball illustrates the body's agency. But we couldn't do this without being attuned to the world through our body. Our senses, such as sound and sight, bring our surroundings to life, and sensations of pleasure and pain also instruct us about our environment. Touch a hot stove and you'll understand how your body informs you of danger!

Body-as-object means that our body is also the means by which things are done to us. We're knocked off our bike, and we fall to the ground. And like all other physical things, we're perceivable by others. We find ourselves judged: too thin, too fat, too short, too tall, and so on. Many girls and people socialized as girls internalize the perspective of others on their body: They objectify themselves. Even if they did not experience this sexualization early in their life, as might be the case for some trans women, eventually many if not all women will feel the weight of the male gaze. And when our body is judged by others, we're sometimes met with disapproval. To avoid this censure, we manage our body: We diet and comply with other beauty standards. The comfort of fitting in and self-objectification go hand in hand. But as we learned in chapter 3, the increasing pressure to look pretty by a specific, narrow standard implies that it's becoming harder to disentangle ourselves from beauty and diet culture. If this is the case, what can we do?

This chapter examines how we can we resist the allure of self-objectification. We'll look at memoirs and philosophical texts that bring the power of movement to the fore. We'll also see how to consider our different bodily abilities when recommending physical activity as a solution to excessive self-objectification. That's why we'll pause at the end to study what I've called "restorative practices"—activities that aren't necessarily athletic but ask us, instead, to focus on what our body feels like from the inside, as opposed to how it looks in the mirror.

The Power of Movement

Before we dive into memoirs that show how reconnecting with our body's capacity for movement can help undo self-objectification, here are a few things to keep in mind. First, I want to emphasize that movement is *one* avenue among many: Some people may not find physical practices empowering. In my experience, intuitive eating and learning to cook were more important forms of self-care than practicing physical exercise. Having said that, valuing the body for its functionality might be helpful to you. Second, I have in mind physical movement that is not exclusively performed for weight loss—we all already know that we can whittle and sculpt our physique through exercise. Instead, I want to underline the connection between confidence in our physical abilities and self-confidence. Third, I also want to leave to the side cases of "compulsive exercise." Psychologists say such exercise is "characterized by a craving for physical training, resulting in uncontrollable excessive exercise behavior with harmful consequences, such as injuries and impaired social relations."[1] I'm excluding compulsive exercise so that we can better explore movement as resistance to beauty culture and, in particular, diet culture. It would be unwise to champion one compulsion (exercise) as a replacement for another compulsion (food restriction)!

Our first stop is Simone de Beauvoir's memoir *The Prime of Life*. We met Beauvoir in chapter 2, where we considered her account of how young girls *become* women, in part, by becoming aware of the male gaze, and the objectification this introduces in their lives. Here, let's have a look at her personal adventures in the Mediterranean Alps in the 1930s. At the time, Beauvoir was a high school philosophy teacher in Marseille, France. On her days off, she often went on hours-long hikes in the neighboring mountains. After her teenage years in Paris, she found freedom and joy in walking and clambering over rocky alpine terrain: "I had never practiced any sport, and therefore took all the more pleasure in driving my body to the very limit of its endurance."[2] Throughout her narrative, she describes the thrill of discovering her body's physical capacities and the feelings of self-confidence that her strenuous walking regime brought. To borrow an expression that has gained currency in feminist circles, Beauvoir's walking provides an example of *embodied resistance*. She cultivated a way of experiencing her body in a world that primarily understood women's bodies through a reductive and objectifying lens.

Although she does not mention her personal experience directly, we find similar insights in her theoretical work. In *The Second Sex*, Beauvoir contrasts boys' and girls' development. Of boys, she writes, "Climbing trees, fighting with his companions, confronting them in violent games, he grasps his body as a means to dominate nature and as a fighting tool; he is proud of his muscles."[3] Of girls, she says, "She is treated like a living doll, and freedom is denied her: thus a vicious circle is closed; for the less she exercises her freedom to understand, grasp, and discover the world around her, the less she will find its resources, and the less she will dare to affirm herself as a subject."[4] Beauvoir is explaining that boys identify with the freedom that physical activities afford. To put things differently, they conceive of their bodies *as subjects*. In contrast, because girls are not encouraged to move as much, they default into feeling like dolls. That is, they experience their bodies *as objects*. Beauvoir adds that this lack of bodily confidence could undermine their overall self-confidence: "To lose confidence in one's body is to lose confidence in one's self."[5]

How relevant are Beauvoir's ideas today? After all, her hikes were in the 1930s and *The Second Sex* was published in 1949. Let's leap to 2025 and the writer and weightlifter Casey Johnston, whose views on intuitive eating were mentioned in the previous chapter. In her memoir *A Physical Education*, she recounts how she engaged in punitive running routines and calorie restriction before discovering the rewards of strength training. As her caloric demands increased with her lifting regimen, her attitude toward food evolved. She began to see it as a source of energy to enjoy rather than one to be restricted. The most significant element of her book is the shift in her attitude about her body. "Before lifting, I had not once thought of myself, my body, as a mutable, habitable living thing. I had not even really thought of myself *as* my body. It was as if it had been a separate, unruly alien entity that I had to wrangle into submission . . . only to find it always falling short."[6] Johnston's "physical education" unfolded at two levels. Concretely, she learned new ways of using her body. Figuratively, her relationship with her body became unified. Instead of a split between her mind and her body, with her mind seeking to micromanage her appearance through diet and cardio, her body became her self. This evolution might remind you of the mind-body and control axes discussed in connection with Susan Bordo's philosophy in chapter 4. For Bordo, many anorectics and bulimics feel a division between mind and body, with the mind seeking to dominate the body. Johnston's training helped her bridge this division and relinquish her need to control her size and shape. To return to the language of self-objectification: She felt her body as a subject, one capable of mastering increasingly difficult physical challenges, while her sense of her body-as-object receded from view.

Beauvoir's and Johnston's memoirs may inspire us to move for the sake of moving, not for the sake of appearance. So should we all start hiking or weightlifting? Doesn't such a recommendation exclude those for whom movement may be difficult? To answer these questions, let's explore the activist Sonya Renee Taylor's book *The Body Is Not an Apology*. Its thesis is simple yet powerful: Because of forms of oppression such as sexism, racism, ageism, ableism, homophobia, and transphobia, many people live in shame about their body and feel the need to apologize for it. Taylor describes a friend with cerebral palsy who suspected she was pregnant. Taylor asks her friend why she didn't use condoms if she didn't want to have a baby. Her friend responds that she did not want to cause any "extra" worries because sex with her disability already felt complicated. To this, Taylor replies: "Your body is not an apology."[7] This sentence later helped Taylor grapple with her own body shame. In her words: "Living in a female body, a Black body, an aging body, a fat body, a body with mental illness is to awaken daily to a planet that expects a certain set of apologies to already live on our tongues."[8] Instead of apologizing for our body, Taylor calls on us to reclaim *radical self-love*. This is a love we were born with. Who hasn't seen a baby delight in their body? The joy they have discovering their fingers and toes. Oppression undoes this love to the point that we feel the need to apologize for our body.

The Body Is Not an Apology provides tools for reclaiming this self-love. One of them, "Be in Movement," bears on our topic.[9] This comes with a twist that Taylor illustrates through her experience. She once felt compelled to take up running and train for a 5K. But because of her body's shape, she often felt discomfort, especially in her breasts. Two weeks into her training, Taylor recognized that running was not for her, and instead of "pushing through her pain," as our culture often tells us to do, she sought a new practice. What was a better fit for her? A West African dance called Moribayassa. "[I] dropped the jogging and found some movement that made me happy."[10] The lesson Taylor takes from this is twofold: Movement can be an act of self-love, but we must also enjoy it. Doing what others tell us is good for our body will backfire if we don't appreciate the recommended form of exercise. Movement can be valuable, but it must be adapted to fit our physical capacities. Taylor's choice of Moribayassa is also telling. She mentions that it's a dance "for women overcoming great adversity."[11] Moribayassa held a deeper significance for a Black woman like Taylor, who is fighting racism and sexism, than it might for someone of a different race or gender simply doing it for fun.

Taylor's switch from running to dancing provides an example of *intuitive exercise*. Connie Sobczak, co-founder of The Body Positive nonprofit, underlines the significance of choosing nurturing movement: "As with learning to eat intuitively, finding exercise that is right for your particular body and life circumstances is a process of trial and error. . . . Our bodies are all made differently and prefer different types of movement. Some people feel better in water, others on land; some feel better doing slow movement, others with vigorous exercise."[12]

Sobczak stresses that sustainability is paramount. Just as dieting often comes with weight-cycling, exercise regimens that don't suit us are bound to backfire. For her, choosing "physical activity that is sustainable throughout our lifetime is the goal, as well as the key to increasing longevity and reducing risk factors for disease."[13]

In the previous chapter, I framed intuitive eating as a form of self-care. Based on Sobczak's analysis, we can also include intuitive exercise. To achieve bodily health and mental well-being, we need to avoid what she calls "all-or-nothing approaches to both eating and exercise."[14] Seeking activities that we enjoy and that accommodate our physical capacities teaches us to become attuned to ourselves from the inside out. In that way, we can learn that our body is more than an object. Punishing our body through physical activity doesn't help us resist self-objectification. Intuitive exercise does.

We lose sight of the power of bodily practices when we construe movement narrowly. Movement can be democratized. So how can we achieve this? Navigating the landscape of a city, let alone a gym or another formal exercise space, can be a challenge for those who live in "minority bodies," a term used by philosopher Elizabeth Barnes to refer to disability. "Being disabled is . . . a way of being a minority with respect to one's body, just as being gay is a way of being a minority with respect to sexuality," Barnes writes.[15] She emphasizes that being disabled "makes you different from the majority, but that difference isn't by itself a bad thing."[16] For Barnes, *ableism* is the root issue. Ableism, in her words, "encompasses more than just personal attitudes—it can include the way our society is structured and organized."[17] These two factors can interact: People who have ableist attitudes may not acknowledge the need to make our physical environments more accessible. But the converse is also true: Those who acknowledge the importance of changing our physical landscapes can contribute to making the shift toward more accessible spaces. Here I have in mind a personal example. For several years, my father, who is sighted, participated in a program where he rode a tandem bike with blind people so they could experience the pleasure of bicycling. In a world free of ableism—not merely as an attitude of individuals, but as a reflection of the structure of our environment—embracing movement could be an option made more welcoming and empowering. Again, this is not to say that everyone should embrace exercise as resistance to self-objectification—we all have our preferences. Instead, let's pay attention to both the meaning of physical activity for people in different bodies and the need to create environments where people can feel free to embrace the type of intuitive movement that's right for them.

Beauvoir's, Johnston's, and Taylor's experiences reflect a claim made by the feminist philosopher Iris Marion Young in her groundbreaking 1980 essay "Throwing Like a Girl." As its title suggests, Young draws on the common phrase, often used as an insult by men, to explore the unique features of girls' and women's physicality. For instance, she notes that we often hold ourselves back during movements that require projecting ourselves into the world, such as throwing a ball or running to catch something. We enact what she calls an "inhibited intentionality," where our body simultaneously affirms an "I can" and an "I cannot."[18] This hesitancy affects how we experience the spaces surrounding us. Whereas a man hops from stone to stone while crossing a stream and doesn't give his steps a second thought, a woman will question whether her footing is sure enough. This creates a dual sense of space: There is a "here" located in our body, and a "yonder" that feels beyond our reach.[19] Toward the end of her essay, Young wonders whether girls' and women's lack of bodily self-confidence could spill over into other areas of their lives: "I have an intuition that the general lack of confidence that we frequently have about our cognitive or leadership abilities is traceable in part to an original doubt of our body's capacity."[20] The stories we've considered show that movement can shape us in ways that surpass the physical and encompass our whole selves.

What Does Science Say About Movement?

Empirical research on exercise validates the links between embracing movement, resisting self-objectification, and gaining confidence in oneself. In *Body Image*, Sarah Grogan presents findings on reducing body dissatisfaction and explains that "self-efficacy" predicts positive body image. She defines self-efficacy as "personal confidence to engage successfully in a specific behavior or succeed in a specific situation" and adds that "it has been suggested that those who feel greater physical self-efficacy are likely to be more body-satisfied."[21] Of particular interest to us is her claim that "self-efficacy may protect college-aged women from disordered eating and negative body image."[22] To back these points, she cites research from the 2010s and a systematic review of thirty-four studies to argue that "there is a growing body of evidence that moderate exercise/physical activity, focusing on physical self-efficacy rather than aesthetics, can improve body satisfaction."[23]

Renee Engeln's work on girls and women adds further support to these ideas. In *Beauty Sick*, Engeln argues that an effective strategy for improving body image lies in valuing the body for its functionality.[24] She cautions that our environment and language around exercise complicate this claim. For example, the mirrors in gyms and expressions like "burning off calories" or working for a "bikini body" can turn exercise into another tool for weight loss. In her survey of women who take group fitness classes, she found that many participants felt self-conscious about instructor comments focused on beauty and body size. On the flip side, "group fitness instructors significantly overestimated the extent to which women in their classes were motivated by appearance."[25] Engeln believes that the instructors' attitudes reinforce the connection between movement and body aesthetics, while neglecting the possibility that exercise could mean something different for their clients. "We're much better off focusing on how exercise makes us feel instead of how it makes us look," she concludes.[26]

Research on athletes vs. non-athletes tells us about the ties between exercise and body image. Let's focus on a 2023 review and meta-analysis of earlier studies on this connection. The paper's premise was that "engaging in sports can increase body appreciation and body functionality (and improve body image), since individuals appreciate their own bodies for how they function, rather than how they look."[27] The authors acknowledge that the issue is made more complex by gender, the expected body type for the sport (lean vs. non-lean), weight requirements, the level of competition, and other factors. For example, they observe that women rugby players "positively interpreted their body shape (strong, muscular) during matches as a tool for performance (athletic body image). However, they felt their athletic bodies failed to meet feminine beauty standards of Western society (social body image)."[28] Take the Olympian rugby player Ilona Maher, well-known for using her platform to promote body positivity. In 2025 Maher declared, "Here I am with yet another gentle but firm reminder that it is OK to exist in a bigger body," before adding that "a lot of us are not meant to be small."[29] Her words capture the tension between her positive experience of her body through sports, her muscular build as a part of her success, and the pressure faced by those who aren't thin. According to the study's authors, "The most robust finding was that athletes have lower levels of body image concerns than non-athletes."[30] I hope that more research will be done to understand how different variables affect this conclusion and to formulate recommendations for coaches of competitive athletes.

The scientific studies suggest that exercise can be a vehicle for self-transformation and resistance to self-objectification. For those of us outside the realm of competitive sports, we can transform and resist if we perform movement for its own sake, or, to put things more colloquially, "for the hell of it," instead of as a way to shrink our bodies, all the while factoring in what's best given our physical abilities. As we saw in chapter 3, the body becomes the self in beauty culture. But the body can also become the self through movement. The difference lies in how we relate to our bodies. When we reduce bodies to their appearance in the eyes of others, we limit ourselves. We're beholden to expectations about which bodies *look good* and which do not. When we develop a different relationship to our body through movement, we define our body *for ourself*. We choose which activities *feel good* and which do not.

The Inner Body and the Promise of Restorative Practices

In *The Body Is Not an Apology*, Taylor also recommends meditation as a tool for cultivating self-love.[31] Although she focuses on mantras, that is, phrases repeated to help focus the mind, meditation in its varied forms can involve the body in movement. Yoga may come to mind. Or walking meditation. This practice involves moving at a slow pace, while coordinating our breath with the rise and fall of our legs and feet, and attending to the minute movements of our body. As one foot lands, we focus on the sensation of the heel striking the ground, then the midfoot meeting that surface, and then the toes grazing it before propelling us into our next step. How should we conceive of our relationship to our body in moments like these?

Let's take a closer look at the connection between attending to these movements and resisting self-objectification. From philosophy, we've learned that the body can be conceived as both a subject and an object. We experience our bodies as centers of subjectivity, but also as things that are "things" open to the scrutiny of others. One of the main components of body-as-a-subject is the notion of *agency*. We act on the world through our body, as we've seen in the previous sections. Being a subject also involves *awareness*. Through our body, we become aware of our surroundings—the table in front of us, the dog barking in the distance, and so on. This is a topic we'll take up in chapter 10. But we're also aware of our own body through our own body! This form of awareness—referred to as *proprioception*—deserves special attention. Proprioception gives us a sense of our body's movements and position without reference to external cues, such as visual ones. For example, if you're scratching an itch on your neck, you draw on proprioception: You're not attending to the specific movements necessary to scratch, and you don't need to think about where your neck is with respect to your other body parts. Using this insight, I'll call the body *as we are aware of it from the inside* "the inner body." In contrast, "the outer body" refers to our body as we perceive it from the outside through our senses. When we look at our legs to see if we have a thigh gap, we perceive our outer body. But when we notice sensations such as tension in our legs, we connect with our inner body.

As someone who has practiced walking meditation, I know how helpful it can be to tune out critical commentary about our bodies and focus on the sensations they afford. One way to situate this activity, as I've practiced it, is under the umbrella of "mindfulness." This is a term for a form of meditation popularized in the West that involves cultivating a non-judgmental awareness, often of the body, from the inside. Jon Kabat-Zinn, a pioneer in the field of research on mindfulness and stress reduction, writes that the awareness developed in mindfulness practices is meant to be non-judgmental.[32] If our mind wanders to the workday during the practice of mindful breathing, we're encouraged to return to our awareness of our breath without beating ourselves up for our digressions. Similarly, when we're engaging in walking meditation, we return to the feelings of our feet and legs whenever we catch ourselves thinking about another topic. In *The Mindful Path to Self-Compassion*, clinical psychologist Christopher K. Germer highlights the link between this form of meditation and the body. He characterizes mindfulness as "a special type of awareness that can keep us anchored safely in our bodies when the going gets tough."[33] Mindfulness does not mean emptying the mind. Rather, it implies providing the mind with an anchor, such as the breath or sensations of comfort or discomfort.[34] Germer indicates that mindfulness can benefit us by helping us cope with painful moments: "When we're mindful, there's less need to escape unpleasant experience—there's a little breathing room around it."[35] Mindfulness puts us in relationship to our inner body.

William Edelglass, a scholar of Buddhism, writes that the term "mindfulness" usually translates the Sanskrit term "smrti,"[36] which refers to our capacity to "sustain focused attention." It is closely allied to the term "samprajanya," which refers to an awareness that "enables the mind to refocus when distracted."[37] A wide range of practices—from breathing exercises to meditations where we express compassion for others—fall under "mindfulness." Yet they all start with cultivating awareness through noticing what's going on in our body. While mindfulness has been promoted as a tool for stress reduction, one overlooked virtue of the practice is that it helps us become of aware of situations that call for a moral response. Jay Garfield clarifies that when we live in distracted, mindless states, we cannot attend to others.[38] Nor can we pay attention to ourselves when we're swept up in the rush of life. Could we include the harms of objectifying ourselves and others on the list of things mindfulness could help us address?

Anchoring ourselves in our body through forms of meditation, such as mindfulness of our breathing or physical sensations, offers a way back to ourselves—one that transcends our appearance. We're *restored* to our body. Meditation, unlike sports, might be made more accessible to people of varying physical abilities, and could furnish an underappreciated means to resist self-objectification. Meditating doesn't appeal to all people, just as cooking, hiking, weightlifting, or dancing doesn't excite everyone. Still, this discipline can teach us how to live in our body in a fuller way than we're expected to do. As Germer puts it, "We live in a body, so to appreciate the fullness of life we need to experience the body."[39] We're taught to adapt our body to dominant beauty standards, and there's safety in complying. It's dangerous to go rogue and to "eff your beauty standards," as one fat activist, Tess Holliday, says. It's also risky to distance ourselves from beauty overall and appreciate our inner body. But what joys may we find when we take that risk?

Fall 2022. I've been in counseling for two years. My weekly sessions with Dalit and cooking lessons with my mother have taught me to appreciate food. The idea that eating normal portions means failure has ebbed. I no longer fear nights like the one that brought me back to my work with Dalit. Progress on my body image issues, however, is slower. Putting on weight—the inevitable outcome of eating more—still bothers me.

I find a solution once I move to a new apartment building. My previous places in Miami both had pools, but I used them infrequently. This time,

I decide to take advantage of a luxury none of the other cities I've lived in have afforded. I begin swimming laps on non-teaching days. Most afternoons, the pool is empty, and I let myself glide undisturbed from end to end. At times, when there is no one in view, I indulge in floating and splashing in the water. I've become enchanted with dolphins since seeing them along the water in my neighborhood. Perhaps inspired, too, by their freedom when I see them leap and play in the bay.

I keep to a slow pace and lose sight of the idea that I'm exercising. I'm not looking to lose weight or even grow muscle. My only aesthetic hope is that stretching my body through the water will help improve my posture. Too much sitting at my computer and too much walking bent over little Carol have left me with slouching shoulders.

After twenty minutes, I dry off in the sun. I don't let myself linger much longer. I want to leave enlivened, not beaten by the heat. Back in my apartment, I shower off the chlorine. I bypass my bathroom mirror before I step into the shower and after, when I towel myself. I don't linger over my thigh gap, my bikini bridge, nor my rib cage. They no longer have any allure . . .

9

Sensualism

Reigniting Pleasure and Desire In and For the Body

> A consequence of female self-love is that the woman grows convinced of social worth. Her love for her body will be unqualified. . . . If a woman loves her own body, she doesn't grudge what other women do with theirs; if she loves femaleness, she champions its rights.
>
> —NAOMI WOLF, *The Beauty Myth*

David greets me in the dark waiting area at the Massage Envy in my neighborhood. Tablet in hand, he guides me to the room where I'll receive my treatment. We sit face-to-face as he reviews the areas that I want him to massage during our hour-long session. "Focus on my shoulders and neck, but cover my whole body. Use medium pressure," I say. I'm easy to please, I think to myself.

He exits, and the second the door shuts behind him, I slip off my tank top and shorts. I then fold and place my clothes in a neat pile on the chair that's by the mirror. I'm mindful not to look at my naked body. Still, I take note that the mirror is shaped like a narrow, wavy band. At best, someone can make sure that their clothes are on all right. But this is not a mirror made for contemplating—let alone criticizing—one's body.

I lie face down on the table and fold the warm blanket over my back. There are few things I look forward to more than a good massage. Since puberty, my relationship with my body has largely been visual. My "body checking" sessions have all unfolded in front of the mirror: thigh-gap check, rib-cage check, no-flesh-folding-over-my-waistband check. But I don't worry that David will check my body. My love of massages comes from a place of trust: I have always believed—I hope not naively—that the therapist does not judge my body. When they pull the blanket from around my head and fold it over my lower back, I don't imagine that they're sweeping their eyes up and down my body, ready to pull out a tape measure to size my waist or my hips. Their task is not to tell me that I should model. The parameters of the transaction are clear.

Still, I can't help but get stuck in my head from time to time. Over the many years I've indulged in massages, I've found myself wondering if my therapist finds my back too bony or my body too thin. With David, I've asked myself if he can notice any changes in my body as I put on weight during recovery. But the thoughts are fleeting. He tells me to breathe in and out three times as he lays a warm, wet towel over my upper back. He lets it linger before wiping my body with soft, slow motions. I hear two squirts from a pump, the tap of his steps as he moves from his station to the table, and then the squishing sounds of massage oils pressed from hand to hand. His fingers land lightly against my back, and I feel liquid swirls against my shoulder blades. I breathe in and catch the scent of citrus.

Minute by minute, the feeling of his hands pressing into my shoulder blades goes from pleasurable to painful. My upper back has never been muscular, and I usually begin to squirm, even with medium pressure, during this portion of the massage. I remind myself to inhale deeply, to take in the pain, and release it through my breath.

The swirls move further down. Down and up. Down and up. And then they stop for a second. I now feel David's fingers press firmly into my lower back. I don't mind the pressure anymore. After kneading my lower back for some time, there is another pause. This time, I feel his elbow touch my torso and then, the weight of his body on mine. I love the wide circles that he draws with his elbow: his coarse arm hair blends with the massage oils, as if, instead of using his arms, he were painting my back with long brushstrokes.

The room is dark, and I keep my eyes tightly shut. I'm reclaiming the inner relationship with my body that I've yearned for since I began writing about body image. My writings speak of cultivating an internal, sensual relationship with one's body. But until I started regular massages, it all sounded theoretical—a connection to one's body would be good to have, but one that I struggled to embody in practice.

Around the time I begin my massage routine, I find myself listening to The Mamas & the Papas' song "Midnight Voyage." They sing, "All aboard, all ashore, at your leisure, take a pleasure trip." I hum the lyrics to myself when I'm walking to and from the bus stop during my commute to school. Having a massage is one of the closest ways I can come to enjoying a "pleasure trip."

IN CHAPTER 4, we discussed the concept of *bodily alienation*—when we're alienated from our body, we mainly experience it from the outside. Our body is no longer our home. Instead, it becomes a foreign thing that we feel compelled to shape and shrink through beauty practices. How can we undo this alienation? How can we live in closer connection to our body? Specifically, let's ask ourselves: *What can pleasure teach us about resisting beauty and diet culture?* As an answer, I'll recommend living more closely to our bodies, loving them in their sensual nature—a philosophy I call *sensualism*. To dig into my response to the unhealthy messaging of diet culture, we'll look at antidotes to bodily alienation, define what pleasure is, and consider how self-objectification affects sexual pleasure. Our whirlwind tour through philosophical conversations about pleasure will teach us the value of undoing bodily alienation and reclaiming bodily integrity.

An Antidote to Bodily Alienation

One of the most prominent philosophers to have described alienation in general is Karl Marx, the nineteenth-century Prussian thinker known for his criticisms of capitalism. The context he discussed in his philosophy was the workplace. In his *Economic and Philosophical Manuscripts of 1844*, he writes that under the capitalist labor conditions, workers felt estranged from four features of their labor: the objects they make; how they're made; their very essence as creative individuals; and their relationships with other people. As an illustration, consider a man hired on a production line to make laptops. Because he can't afford the computers he is assembling, Marx would claim, "the object confronts him as something hostile and alien."[1] If the man were living in privileged circumstances, he would instead be using the laptop. He also has no ownership over the method of creating the machine; it's all a soulless routine that he has no say in. This situation eats at him. Why? For Marx, creative activity is essential to us as people, and to dictate its parameters crushes us. It alienates us. Lastly, under these labor conditions, we can't help but feel estranged from others, in particular, those who are running the show.

What would a life free from alienation look like? In another work, "Excerpts from James Mill's Elements of Political Economy," Marx depicts "unalienated labor." Under new conditions—ones where we express our creativity and have autonomy in our productive activities—our "work would be a free manifestation of life, hence an enjoyment of life."[2] This sentence has much to teach us about transforming bodily alienation. Just as the unalienated worker would enjoy his work, so too, under different conditions, would we *enjoy* our bodies. How would we feel if we weren't alienated?

To fill in this picture, let's circle back to the four elements of alienation in the workplace. First, Marx thought that we're alienated from the objects we make. While the body is not something we create from scratch ourselves, we do creatively contribute to what it becomes through our choices around what we put into our bodies and what we do with our bodies. If we were free to enjoy our bodies, we might try to shape them in liberating ways or not seek to alter them at all. We would not feel pressured to shrink ourselves or otherwise fit beauty standards. For example, someone who thrives on weightlifting might engage in the exercise to sculpt their body, but they may also adopt the practice for its own sake—for the sheer satisfaction of lifting heavier and heavier things.

Second, Marx worried that laborers couldn't express themselves because they were hamstrung by the workplace's organization—for instance, the structure of assembly lines. Enjoying our bodies would mean having the freedom to engage in the movements that energize us. We could choose *how* to use our bodies. Sonya Renee Taylor's story about switching from running to dancing would be an example of this kind of freedom.

Third, what's fundamental to us as human beings, according to Marx, is our creative labor—something that's quashed under capitalism. How could we transpose this idea to the body? In a society emancipated from rigid beauty standards, we could make what we want of our bodies: create new aesthetic standards, reject the ones that hurt us, or even opt out of beauty culture altogether.

Fourth, the workplace, as it's often configured, creates hierarchies and sometimes animosity between people of the same rank (who can best compete for the boss's recognition?). In a freer world, we would not feel hostility toward one another based on our appearance. To paraphrase Naomi Wolf, a woman who loves her own body doesn't judge what other women do with theirs. We wouldn't rank people based on their looks, we wouldn't feel body shame, and we wouldn't feel like failures in the eyes of others.

Notice the "we" in these statements. For Marx, to create the conditions to enjoy labor, workers must unite and overthrow capitalism. This is not our concern here. What we need to do is challenge beauty culture, especially diet culture—many women derive their self-worth from looking beautiful, and one of the most corrosive beauty standards is extreme thinness. I'll return to the problem of collective action later in this chapter.

I want to define an unalienated relationship with our bodies as one of enjoyment. To enjoy our bodies, we need to be closely attuned to them from the inside, to embrace their sensual nature. This is *sensualism*. Our bodies are not just objects to behold and to mold. To the contrary. They can be sources of pleasure.

Living for Pleasure

Pleasure, one of the many sensations our bodies afford, directs so much of what we do, so let's have a closer look at it.* In the history of philosophy, very generally, there are two prominent views, which I refer to as the simple picture and the complex picture. According to the simple picture, pleasure is "a single simple (feature of) experience that makes experiences good and attractive to the extent it is present."[3] Just as the redness of an apple is a simple feature of experience when I look at it, so too with pleasure. What's distinctive of pleasure is that it's intrinsically good. The redness of the apple is value-neutral, whereas its sweet taste is positive. Different objects can cause pleasure: the sweetness of milk chocolate, the smell of a rose, loving touch, and so on. Here, there seems to be a unity of experience: "On the simple picture, pleasure itself is always the same; when it is bound up with the different pleasures of sweets or philosophy it is only *caused* . . . in different ways."[4]

Philosophers quibble with the simple picture for many reasons, one of which is that there seems to be little in common between the pleasures that various objects give us. Is the pleasure of chocolate commensurable with the ecstasy of an orgasm? Perhaps it's better to characterize pleasure in terms of motivation. Consider the English utilitarian Henry Sidgwick, another nineteenth-century philosopher, who thought that trying to single out agreeable moments through introspection is not good enough to identify pleasure. Instead, we need to account for how objects drive our attention and actions. In this complex picture, something counts as pleasurable—chocolate, a rose, touch—if we're drawn to the object or seek it out.

There's something intuitive about this picture because many objects affect us in more varied ways than the simple picture seems to allow. For example, someone may speak of a "pleasurable morning"—a way of singling out an extended period of relaxation or ease. This

* The title of this section is borrowed from Emily Austin's book on Epicurus, *Living for Pleasure: An Epicurean Guide to Life* (Oxford University Press, 2023).

expression needn't imply having a series of simple pleasures: eating chocolate, smelling a rose, and then feeling a loving touch. We're not saying that we had a morning with a critical mass of discrete pleasures; rather, we're saying that our general experience of the morning as a whole was pleasant. By contrast, during a stressful morning, while we might have a bite of chocolate, we cannot always be said to savor it. We wolf it down without having genuinely tasted it. We might go so far as to say that there was no pleasure, even if we tasted the chocolate. During the stressful morning, our attention is so fixed on other matters that we don't attend to the same chocolate that once had such a tasty flavor.

The proponent of the more complex view would say that we need to take into consideration how our attention affects enjoyment. Instead of opposing these pictures, though, I want to combine them. Perhaps there is an "experiential core" to pleasure, even if we use the concept in loose ways—sometimes to refer to the sensations arising from things, sometimes to the ambiance that makes possible such sensations.

Some philosophical traditions view sensual pleasure with suspicion. Epictetus, a philosopher from the Stoic school, advised: "If you are struck by the appearance of any promised pleasure, guard yourself against being hurried away by it."[5] We should analyze objects and evaluate the pleasure they may provide before pursuing them. Marcus Aurelius, also a Stoic, went so far as to say that "no [good] man would ever repent of having refused any sensual pleasure. Pleasure then is neither good nor useful."[6] While Stoics didn't reject enjoyment, they regarded pleasure as an "indifferent"—something outside our control. As such, it wasn't the highest good in life. Above all, they valued virtues, such as temperance, which, in Marcus Aurelius's words, "is opposed to love of pleasure."[7]

But not all schools mistrust pleasure. When discussing self-care in chapter 7, I also referred to the ancient Greek philosopher Epicurus, who said that "pleasure is the alpha and omega of a happy life."[8] His view would fit under simple picture since he defines pleasure as "the absence of pain in the body and of trouble in the soul."[9] Anything that satisfies this definition counts as pleasure. Epicurus cautions that not all pleasures are worth pursuing: "Since pleasure is our first and native good, for that reason we do not choose every pleasure whatever, but often pass over many pleasures when a greater annoyance ensues from them."[10] Instead, he favors simple pleasures: "Bread and water confer the highest possible pleasure when they are brought to hungry lips."[11] We can find fulfillment in satisfying our basic needs. So his position resembles the Stoics': We shouldn't chase every enjoyment. Nevertheless, there's a different emphasis in these competing schools. Among philosophers in the Western tradition, Epicurus stands out: The body is not an appendage whose desires we need to control with a tight fist—fulfilling the body's wants and developing tranquility of mind can both be sources of happiness. Stoics view the pursuit of pleasure as a threat to our peace of mind, while Epicureans think of pleasure as a good so long as we cultivate it in moderation.

A final point related to the problem of body image: The physical pleasures Epicurus has in mind are not those of beautification. In part 1, we learned of the pleasure derived from creating new looks or from contemplating our bodies, and I mentioned the joys of makeup and fashion. But as we saw, these can also harm us. When we go to extreme lengths to change our appearance, we can jeopardize our physical health. Not so with Epicurean pleasures. When chosen wisely, and moderated accordingly, Epicurean pleasures do not harm us the way beauty standards do.

Another tradition that emphasizes pleasure is Tantra. This philosophy and religion, originating in Hinduism and Buddhism, ties enlightenment to enjoyment. As the Tibetan monk Lama Thubten Yeshe describes it, "Instead of advocating separation from worldly pleasures the way many other traditions do, tantra empathizes that it is much more effective for humans to enjoy themselves and channel the energy of their enjoyments into a quick and powerful path to fulfillment and enlightenment."[12] Lama Yeshe writes that it's our "grasping and attachment" to pleasures that causes problems, not the pleasures themselves.[13] According to him, we mistakenly blame objects for our unhappiness. If we're disappointed with our partner's looks, we crave a more attractive person. If we're disappointed with our car, we crave a newer and faster one.[14] We place unreasonable expectations on things to secure happiness. When one thing disappoints us, we seek a replacement, and if this replacement disappoints, we seek yet another replacement. For him, tantric practice puts an end to this seeking by training us to reject the duality that casts one object as deficient and its successor as better. Tantra harnesses "the same desirous energy that ordinarily propels us from one unsatisfactory situation to another."[15] What we achieve is "a transcendental experience of bliss and wisdom."[16] Although the final aims of Epicureanism and Tantra differ, again, the goal is not to find pleasure in the "outer body," but rather to become aware of the pleasures arising in us.

"Religion," in an etymological sense, signifies reconnecting. The word likely derives from the Latin "religare": "to bind fast."[17] This etymology hints at the idea that religion is a way of fastening us to something, to some source. The link between physical pleasure and enlightenment in Tantra suggests that reconnecting to our bodies may guide us to something greater than our mundane concerns, including those about our physiques. Inspired by this tradition, I'm suggesting that we embrace the inner body through physical pleasures. Instead of obsessing over our appearance and trying to change it through diet, exercise, cosmetic procedures, and the like, what if we tuned in to ourselves? Valuing our bodies in their sensual nature is an overlooked source of empowerment, and perhaps even of enlightenment. Like movement, sensuality can help us resist the allure of self-objectification.

Can We Enjoy Sex with Our Body on Our Mind?

Sex is one domain where body image concerns and enjoyment collide. Anecdotes and psychological studies of body image and sexuality show that our external perspective on our own body affects how we experience sexual pleasure.

One story that paints a powerful picture of body dissatisfaction affecting sexual pleasure is writer Jenny Powers's "Outsourcing My Orgasm." Powers describes how self-consciousness about her body prevented her from enjoying sex with her husband. After gaining weight, she began avoiding sex because she couldn't take her mind off her changed body: "Somewhere along the line, I'd let the thoughts in my head take over, and it's hard to have an orgasm when you're too busy wondering if you're positioned in the least fat way possible. . . . Even when masturbating, I couldn't control the strength of my self-degrading thoughts, so I gave up on that, too."[18] At that point, Powers decided to make a change in her life. She sought an erotic massage with a specialized therapist. After experiencing an orgasm thanks to this specialist, she began to initiate sex again and feel less dissatisfied with her body. Of her transformation, she writes, "Now I focus on how my clothes fit instead of what size is marked on the labels."[19] Once more comfortable being naked in her husband's presence, she doesn't "always insist the lights be turned off during sex."[20]

This story makes vivid the research on the relationship between body image and sexual well-being. In a 2019 review of studies exploring this relationship, researchers conclude, "The extant findings suggest that positive body image is associated with a variety of adaptive sexual experiences including safe sex, sexual desire, sexual functioning, communication about sex, and comfort with sex. In contrast, women who experience body dissatisfaction report an increased likelihood of experiencing a variety of negative sexual experiences."[21] Appreciating our appearance doesn't automatically translate into enjoying sex, but this study shows that we're more inclined to speak about safer sexual practices or to share our likes and dislikes—both foundations for a better partnered sex life—when we have a positive self-image.

The tie between body satisfaction and sexual satisfaction also applies to our solo sex lives. According to another study of women's sexuality, different levels of negative or positive body image predicted differing reported levels of sexual pleasure and incidences of orgasm during partnered sex and masturbation. "Body image dissatisfaction and likely concomitant psychological distress are related to impaired orgasmic response during both partnered sex and masturbation and may diminish sexual relationship satisfaction," the authors write.[22] Based on previous research, they also speculate about the causal connections between masturbation and sexual enjoyment: "Women who masturbate are more able to associate sexual pleasure with their bodily responses and, in doing so, develop greater satisfaction with their bodies."[23] Taking this a step further, it's worth asking: Could enjoying one's body *from the inside* teach us to appreciate our whole selves?

Renowned sex educator Emily Nagoski connects the dots between body dissatisfaction and sexual enjoyment with a simple equation: "criticizing yourself = stress = reduced sexual pleasure."[24] According to her, criticizing ourselves about our bodies is a form of stress. "Your body reacts to negative self-evaluations as if you're under attack," she says.[25] "How would it feel to have a person you care about touching you and looking at you, when the thought of your own body makes you uncomfortable? Would you pay attention to the sensations in your body and your partner's—or would you pay attention to all the things you feel compelled to hide?"[26] Nagoski's questions help clarify the relation between sexual pleasure and attention. If we're thinking about what we look like during sex, how can we be present? Dividing our attention between our imagined appearance and sex acts themselves can only dilute our pleasure. Just as checking our phone while savoring a meal is bound to diminish the intensity of our experience, having our appearance on our mind might prevent us from being *in* our body.

Her solution to this problem is "to practice replacing self-criticism with self-kindness."[27] She notes that while women are initially drawn to self-acceptance, they tend to step back because they believe that self-criticism will keep them motivated.[28] Drawing on empirical research, she sketches three paths to self-acceptance. First, we need to develop *self-compassion*. For example, she invites her readers to write a letter about a difficult situation that they're facing, but to write it in the second person ("you") as though they were advising a friend. She notes that we would probably use compassionate language in this case.

So why not do the same for ourselves? Second, to release self-criticism, she recommends creating *cognitive dissonance*—the feeling of discomfort we have when we hold opposing beliefs. According to her, we can achieve this by looking at our body in the mirror and listing what we like about it. Although we'll shrink from our lists at first, the more we do this, the easier it will be to develop "self-appreciating thoughts."[29] Third, she advocates *media nutrition.* We should cull our media feeds of content that "reinforces body self-criticism."[30] The jury is still out about media literacy—for example, Renee Engeln, whose work we've visited several times, expresses skepticism about the effectiveness of warning labels on altered images.[31] Nonetheless, it seems reasonable to minimize our exposure to pictures and videos that make us feel worse about our body.

Is Skinniness a True Pleasure?

"Nothing tastes as good as skinny feels." You might have heard model Kate Moss's controversial quip from a 2009 interview.[32] Moss, who later expressed regret about her statement, said that she first came across it pasted on the fridge of her former housemate and hairdresser, James Brown.[33] The phrase indicates that the feeling of being skinny trumps any food choice you might make. But could the feeling of skinniness—whatever this means—be truly pleasurable? Moss's words raise a philosophical problem with a long history: Is there a real distinction between true and false pleasures? Let's suppose that there is one. Could skinniness be a true pleasure? One even superior to that of food? I doubt this. And if you've read this far, I bet you do, too. But to better answer these questions, let's examine the ancient philosopher Plato's views on false pleasures.

In the *Philebus*, a dialogue featuring his teacher Socrates, we witness a conversation about what makes for a good life.[34] Is it a life of wisdom? Of pleasure? Or both? During this discussion, we learn of the distinction between true and false pleasures. It's obvious that our beliefs about the world can be true or false. If I think that the Eiffel

Tower was built by Egyptians in Antiquity, then I have a false belief. If I think that it was conceived of by the engineers Émile Nouguier and Maurice Koechlin for the 1889 Exposition Universelle, then I have a true belief. So too with pleasures, according to Socrates. For instance, I may relish the champagne that I see the server bringing to me. This anticipatory pleasure becomes falsified, however, when it turns out that the drink is a mediocre prosecco. I don't receive the good I looked forward to. Or I may anticipate being fulfilled by winning the lottery. Suppose that I win it and end up spending the money frivolously, while being plagued by jealous friends and family, and feeling miserable. I anticipated something that I did receive (unlike the champagne case), but it turned out that having a lot of money doesn't make for a good life. These situations concern future objects. What about the present? Can the pleasures we enjoy in the moment be false?

While Socrates's reasoning on this topic is controversial, commentator Patricia Marechal helps clear up some of the confusion. She draws our attention to the dialogue's sections on malice and comedy. There, Socrates asks his interlocutor, Protarchus, "Are you aware that even at a comedy the soul experiences a mixed feeling of pain and pleasure?"[35] In the face of Protarchus skepticism, Socrates responds that finding joy in someone else's misfortunes—as we do in some forms of humor—is a pleasure mixed with pain. Who hasn't laughed at someone's expense? According to Socrates, this is an example of a false pleasure. It's the mark of a vicious character, since a good person shouldn't delight in another person's suffering. The pleasure we take in such forms of comedy isn't worthwhile. Marechal summarizes her interpretation by saying that, for Plato, "pleasures are true when we take them in things that are worthy of enjoyment."[36] Whether present or future, pleasures are true only if the object of pleasure is worth enjoying. The suffering of other people is intrinsically bad, so the pleasure we might take in it is a false pleasure.

Let's bring the Socratic insight back to Moss's quip. Assuming that there is a pleasure in thinness, is it a true pleasure? I don't think so—for the reasons provided in the *Philebus*. Skinniness is not a true pleasure because it's not worthy of our enjoyment. Why? Because this supposed pleasure is founded on the misguided idea that being skinny makes us more valuable human beings. Whatever the pleasure skinniness may afford, it isn't one worthy of our enjoyment, and it's the mark of a flawed character to find fulfillment in it. Of course, dieting to be thin can backfire—either in the form of chronic yo-yo dieting or in the slide to an eating disorder. But what's most relevant here is that the norm of feminine slenderness is bad because of its origins in discrimination. As the genealogy of thinness from chapter 1 highlighted, our prejudice against fatness originates in racist and sexist beliefs. We've also learned that discrimination runs rampant based on sometimes flawed reasoning between health and body size. More than anything, the idea that fat persons are *morally* unworthy is also false. In *Unshrinking*, Kate Manne points out that our moral panic about obesity fails to recognize the social issues—food deserts, infrastructure that discourages physical activity, and poverty—that drive our weight up.[37] We condemn people for their bodies as though gaining weight were merely a matter of "letting oneself go" and caving to wild appetites. True, there's comfort in fitting in by being skinny, but we've long found comfort and acceptance in other morally dubious ideas—and that doesn't make them good. So let's stop equating body size and worth. And let's stop finding pleasure in being thin. It would be wrong to say that *all* things taste better than skinny feels. I doubt many people like the taste of rotten meat, among other disgusting things. But I'm certain of this: Whatever foods delight you taste better than skinny feels!

Sensualism as a Feminist Practice

Marx's philosophy guided us from the problem of bodily alienation to a solution: finding joy in our sensual nature. We've probed this idea by exploring physical pleasure, including sexual enjoyment. His theories can help us further. He argued that workers' solidarity could help undo the conditions that breed their alienation. Can we apply this thesis to the topic of sensualism? In other words, can we make sensualism a collective practice?

We've talked about how difficult it is to break free from beauty culture. Being attractive is not merely about looking a certain way, but also about securing goods, such as dating prospects and job opportunities. Beautification can be an economic calculation. Is it worth spending money on clothes and cosmetics to land a better job? The same can be said of thinness. Our efforts to lose weight—even if they are short-lived—offer a payoff. This creates a problem for changing beauty standards. The more we live up to reigning beauty standards, the more they're normalized, and the harder it becomes to challenge them. Yet I want to show you that this self-reinforcing cycle is not inevitable. It can be beaten with collective action, the same way that some people inspired by Marx achieved reductions in child labor and the length of workweeks, increases in holidays, and the introduction of health benefits for workers and their families.

To increase the odds of overcoming the pressure to be thin, we need to unite. I take this lesson, in part, from the essays included in *Embodied Resistance: Challenging the Norms, Breaking the Rules*. There, Chris Bobel and Samantha Kwan collect essays that prove the power of coming together. In one essay, researchers Breanne Fahs and Denise Delgado trace an experiment that they conducted in a course on women and health. They invited the nineteen women in the class to stop removing body hair for a period of twelve weeks. They found that some of the women who opted out of the experiment felt marginalized by those who took part in it. Conversely, a few women who opted in continued to refrain from shaving even after the experiment was over. The authors summarize their findings in these terms: "Although the original intent of the experiment was to challenge social norms and subvert compulsory shaving demands, the assignment ultimately created a new social norm within the classroom."[38] Not removing body hair became the new body aesthetic, and those who continued to shave ended up being outliers.

In another essay in the volume, "Fat. Hairy. Sexy: Contesting Standards of Beauty and Sexuality in the Gay Community," Nathaniel

C. Pyle and Noa Logan Klein draw on the idea of a "tactical repertoire" to isolate the ways bears, big men, and those attracted to them (sometimes known as "chasers") challenge stereotypes about gay male bodies and sexual attraction—within both queer communities and heterosexual culture. They claim that *solidarity*, *contestation*, and *intentionality* define these challenges. *Solidarity* means that "collective action by a group usually involves a certain degree of collective identity or solidarity and unity around a specific cause. . . . The group must see how they are joined by something that is oppressing them and that acting together to change that structure gives them a certain amount of common ground."[39] *Contestation* implies public display. In the case Pyle and Klein delve into, "socializing in public and semipublic gay and nongay spaces in which non-community members are confronted with their bodies and sexualities forces onlookers to notice their oppositional identities."[40] What they mean, in simpler terms, is that when we see bodies and behaviors that defy our typical representations of attractiveness being proudly displayed, we're challenged to examine our own prejudices. The presence of big men and bears "can have lasting effects on individuals, broadening ideas or perceptions of queer bodies for many whose previous perceptions of gay men were the result of . . . limited media representation."[41] And we can make similar observations about the public displays made by chasers. Just as displaying one's own body when it doesn't conform to dominant beauty standards can be an act of protest, so too displaying one's attraction to bodies outside the norm can be a form of contestation. *Intentionality* refers to the "notion that deliberate forethought informs the contestation of power structures."[42] Basically, for the displays made by big men, bears, and chasers to count as revolutionary, these men must do so with this intent in mind. "Big men, bears, and chasers proudly display their bodies and sexualities as a means to challenge narrow stereotypes of gay male beauty and sexuality," Pyle and Klein say.[43]

Let's now apply these lessons to sensualism. What if adopting this practice could become a new bodily norm—one that would displace the tyranny of thinness? The essays from *Embodied Resistance* show that group norms can be transformed—as in the case of women and body hair removal—or that public displays can defy our stereotypes and transform our understanding of others—as in the case of big men and bear communities. Let's envision a society where, regardless of our size, we enjoy our bodies in their sensual nature. Such countercultures are already in the making. Connie Sobczak, whose ideas on intuitive exercise we touched on in chapter 8, has made a career of organizing groups where people find joy in their bodies, not because they slip into a certain dress size, but rather because of the pleasures they find in movement. That's been the mission of her nonprofit, The Body Positive. And if we circle back to the feminist upheavals of the 1960s and '70s, that's the type of work sex educators like Betty Dodson accomplished when she taught others, especially women, to experience orgasm in her "Bodysex Workshops."[44] This is the activism that we need to resist the domination of thinness.

These changes would help us break out of the self-reinforcing cycle that has elevated slenderness again and again over the past centuries. In my academic work on the thigh gap fetish, I called sensualism a "feminist practice."[45] Why? Because embracing our sensuality is an act of protest in a culture that still puts an undue burden on women to objectify themselves and whittle away their bodies. Sensualism, by its very nature, means resistance to such a culture. Yet people of all genders increasingly feel this objectification burden. So sensualism has a revolutionary potential for all of us. In using the term "feminist practice," I want to remind us of the roots of the slenderness ideal in sexist oppression and to conceive of sensualism as a new ideal for women, one that can be extended as a gift to all.

In October 2022, around the time my weight falls into a "normal" range, I meditate on what it means to perfect oneself and reflect on pleasure's value for personal development. A running theme during counseling has been my perfectionism. As I run through these thoughts, I dive into a longtime favorite—Spinoza's *Ethics*. There, the philosopher says, "Pleasure is the transition of a man from a lesser to a greater perfection." Perfectionism—being the perfect daughter, being perfect for modeling—has driven me to disordered eating. Spinoza also claims that certain emotions, or what he calls "passions," such as fear or lust, enslave us. Since puberty, I've lived with the fear of seeing my weight on the scale rise, of feeling any fat on my body. Since puberty, I've lusted for the thinnest body: the thigh gap, the collarbones, the ribs poking out.

My eating disorder has thrived on these fears and these lusts. It told me that restrictive eating would be for my own benefit. That it would help become a model. That it would make me a good citizen in a society hooked on thinness. As I comb over the *Ethics*, I realize that I've become the disorder's slave.

Spinoza adds that our passions can prevent us from perfecting ourselves. Besides being thin, I've longed to excel as a philosopher and a writer, as a friend, and as a caregiver for my dog, Carol. The more I fear weight gain, the more I distract myself from these projects. And the more I lust for a thin body, the more I drain myself of the strength to pursue my passions. Near the end of the *Ethics*, Spinoza writes that only when we have "clear ideas" about our passions can we live free lives. Reason helps us form these ideas and grasp which of our passions control us. In return, we can take control of them.

If Spinoza is right that "pleasure is the transition of a man from a lesser to a greater perfection," then the modern view of thinness has been a false pleasure. It has diminished me. What real pleasures await me? Two years of counseling have gone by, and I'm beginning to experience them. The delight of eating, the joys of cooking, the peace of sleeping through the night without gnawing hunger, the rush of water as I swim laps in my pool, the fulfillment of walking for hours with Carol.

10

Remaking the World

> Playfulness is, in part, an openness to being a fool, which is a combination of not worrying about competence, not being self-important, not taking norms as sacred and finding ambiguity and double edges a source of wisdom and delight. So, positively, the playful attitude involves openness to surprise, openness to being a fool, openness to self-construction or reconstruction and to construction or reconstruction of the "worlds" we inhabit playfully.
>
> —MARÍA LUGONES, "Playfulness, 'World'-Travelling, and Loving Perception"

I ditch my full-length mirror as I near the end of my second round of eating disorder counseling. I've spent too many years "body checking" to abandon the practice merely by telling myself not to use my mirror. The only way to resist its allure is to get rid of it. My therapist doesn't tell me to do so. None of the online forums for eating recovery advise it. This is my decision alone.

There are interesting analogies and disanalogies between addiction and eating disorder recovery. Unlike an alcoholic or drug addict, we can't address our condition by abstaining from a substance. Neither binge eaters, bulimics, nor anorectics can simply not eat. We need to find a balance between eating too much and too little food. But like those with an addiction, we may need to abandon some practices—at least for a period. Mine is the mirror. My scale was gone by the time I entered my second phase of counseling. I had already had the good sense to get rid of it. But the mirror has remained hanging in my closet.

I take the mirror off its rack and place it outside my apartment door with the word "free" written in all caps on a taped sign.

A friend recently said that I'm a "no-nonsense person." I had never thought of myself in that regard. But she may be on to something. At the airport, an airline check-in agent once told me that my dog was too tall for her carrier and that I might not be able to fly back home with her for Thanksgiving. I was annoyed at him for a moment. But I did not panic, nor did I argue with him or his boss. I was already scheming to buy a ticket on another airline. End of story.

Maybe this attitude explains why I don't feel any anguish when I place the mirror outside my door. I've settled on the most logical course of action, given my issues, and I follow through with it. If anything, I feel relieved. Once I close the door, I go back to my teaching preparations for the coming week. I soon hear rummaging outside.

Ridding myself of the mirror will become one of the best decisions I make as part of my recovery. I cannot easily keep track of the changes in my body as I put on weight. No more body checking. Every few days, I succumb to sneaking a peek at my body in the bathroom mirror. But as a rule, I don't. I step out of the shower and lotion myself with my eyes closed, focusing on massaging it into my skin. I've chosen that lotion because I love its heavy, fruity odor. I luxuriate in the sensations of touch and its fragrance post-shower. Much like in the myth of Orpheus and Eurydice, I know that if I take a glance, I will be dragged back into the underworld.

The only issue with not owning a full-length mirror comes in matters of fashion. I cannot easily determine if my shoes match my outfit. So I swing my legs up in front of my bathroom mirror. That's all. Some acrobatics, no nonsense.

THROUGHOUT THIS BOOK, I've emphasized that the body is a subject. In filling in this claim, I described the significance of the body's movements and the meaning of sensual pleasure. I've focused, in other terms, on our inner relationship to our body. But the body is also our opening onto the *world* and our medium for interacting with it. What is the meaning of the body-world connection? What can it teach us about resisting self-objectification and diet culture? This book's final guiding question will be: *How can we remake the world in more empowering ways?*

Addressing this question will take us through a tour of authors such as Martin Heidegger and María Lugones, and from topics ranging from the act of reading books to walking through nature. We'll look at the structure of cultural worlds, and we'll talk about moving between such worlds. Then we'll explore how to remake cultures, with a focus on diet culture. We'll finish by asking where the natural world fits into revolutionizing our understanding of ourselves and of others.

We've seen that excessive self-objectification is to our detriment. A straightforward solution to it would sound something like this: "Stop thinking about your body! Appreciate the world around you—the light as you watch the sun rise, or the harmonies as you listen to your favorite music." But this response implies a binary that is too simplistic. It sets apart two things—the self and the world—and tells you to only focus on the world. This answer neglects two things: first, that we are part of the world; second, that our bodies are precisely the hinge point through which we inhabit the world. I say "inhabit" deliberately: we can *access* the world through our bodily senses, but we also *create* worlds. An uninhabited house or an empty apartment bears no trace of our personality; it won't until we decorate it. So, too, a world devoid of our bodily activities would not bear witness to our *being* in the world. We stamp the world with our bodies in a literal sense (a footprint, let's say), but we also do so through our ways of using objects, creating them, and sharing them.

What Is a World?

To get a handle on these claims, we first need to ask a daunting question: What is a world? And as daunting as this question is, so too is the person I'm enlisting to help us answer it. His name is Martin Heidegger.

This German philosopher is sometimes praised as the deepest thinker of the twentieth century, sometimes criticized as a charlatan who pretends to be profound by using obscure language. My assessment lies somewhere in the middle. On the one hand, he had significant insights that influenced people like my all-time-favorite philosopher, Simone de Beauvoir. When Heidegger states that the self and the world form a unity, Beauvoir translates this into saying that the body and world are integrated. The body is not just a thing. Rather, it's a "situation"—our "grasp on the world" and the "sketch of our projects."[1] On the other hand, Heidegger complicated matters by creating an idiom that defies many philosophers, especially those unfamiliar with German. Take his definition of a world from his magnum opus *Being and Time*: A world is "that 'wherein' a factical Dasein as such 'lives.'"[2] Good grief! What is "factical"? What is a "Dasein"? What's the significance of putting quotations around "lives"? To bypass these questions, which would require a whole book on *Being and Time*, we can appeal to Heidegger himself. In his lectures to his students on the topic of worlds, he expresses himself in terms that don't require a philosophical lexicon.

In his snail analogy, in lectures gathered under the title *History of the Concept of Time*, Heidegger says, "We can say that the snail at times crawls out of its shell and at the same time keeps it on hand; it stretches itself out to something, to food, to some things which it finds on the ground."[3] If we're like snails, then each of the things we do—reading this book, talking with someone about it, and so on—is a different way of inhabiting the world. Heidegger then asks, "Does the snail thereby first enter into a relationship of being with the world? Not at all! Its act of crawling out is but a local modification of its already-being-in-the-world."[4] His analogy implies that we never exist divorced from a world. There's no "shell" that we retreat into and then leave when we go about our life. Self and world are not opposed to one another. So if the world isn't just a place we get beamed into when we're born and get ejected out of when we die, what's it like? To push the snail analogy, we should ask what's distinctive of our way of being in the world. As snails inhabit their worlds, they do the snail thing—crawling and eating plants. But we do something else with ours. What is this something else?

Think about your experience of reading this book. You're not hallucinating a philosopher's voice. Rather, you're in some posture, such as sitting. You're likely holding a paperback or an e-reader, or perhaps you're driving and listening to an audiobook. For the sake of simplicity, let's say you're in your living room, sitting on a couch, with a paperback version of this book in your hand. You squint as you start this chapter, but then you turn your lamp on to help your eyesight. Once you do that, you get in the flow as you read: You're paying explicit attention neither to the size and shape of the book, nor to your body, nor to your living room. Now suppose you spy a creeping bug out of the corner of your eye. You're not one to let bugs coexist peacefully in your environment. So you start chasing it. After a few swipes, you kill it with this book. You dispose of the bug and settle back on your couch.

This incident reveals essential features of the self-world relationship according to Heidegger. First, our worlds are composed of things that "refer" to one another. The lamp helps you see the book; the couch helps you rest your arm, and so on. They form what Heidegger calls "referential totalities."[5] But referential totalities only exist as they're defined by our purposes. If you want to nap instead of read, then the couch's arm becomes a substitute for a pillow instead of a means to prop your arm. And when you spy that critter, the book is no longer something "in-order-to" read.[6] Rather, it's a tool for killing bugs.

Second, the book is in a language that you comprehend. Otherwise, the pages would be random pieces of paper with undecipherable characters. While you might have learned from others to read in whatever language you're using for this book, the very idea of reading a book is not something you were born with. Instead, people in your family or your school showed you what the purpose of a book was. For Heidegger, the social world is the background that helps us understand the different uses of things.

Third, if you're reading *this* book as opposed to a textbook on geology or a romance novel, it's because you have a stake in what I'm saying.

You, the reader, might identify as a survivor of disordered eating or as a feminist—or both. Such an identity—what Heidegger calls a "for-the-sake-of-which"—is what guides the whole activity.[7] This identity is what got you onto your couch with the book in hand, until the pesky intruder caught your eye. If you identify more as a surfer than a reader, then on a day with good waves, you're at the beach instead of on your couch. Moreover, our identities are social: Being a reader is an identity, so is being an eating disorder survivor, and so is being a feminist. Heidegger thinks of them as "possibilities" for us rather than static features of ourselves.[8]

Putting these three elements together, Heidegger would say that being in a world means: 1) using objects for specific purposes; 2) learning how to use objects thanks to others; 3) adopting identities that are shared with others. These factors all come together to define worlds. Human worlds are, in short, far more complex than snail-plant combinations.

Between Worlds

The "world" isn't just a way of referring to our planet. Rather, if we draw on Heidegger's ideas, worlds are interactive. They bring together inanimate things, such as books and lamps, and tie people to one another through shared activities, such as teaching a child to read, or shared identities, such as being a feminist. "World" is used in a figurative sense, as in the "fashion world" or the "world of academia." Each of these worlds is organized around different settings (runways vs. libraries), objects (clothes hangers vs. books), roles (photographers vs. students), and aspirations (to "get a break" as a model vs. to excel as a teacher).

We aren't locked in our worlds, unlike being bound to the earth by the pull of gravity. When we move through our daily life—let's say, shuttling from home to work and back—we travel between worlds. And when our goals evolve, we can leave worlds behind: for instance, leaving home for college or moving to a new city for a new career. To understand the significance of such "world-traveling," let's consider the feminist thinker María Lugones. We'll be able to combine her ideas with Heidegger's theory and imagine what it takes to *remake* the world. My goal in writing this book has been to inspire us to shape the world in a less oppressive way—one where our value isn't dependent on our body size or our eating habits.

María Lugones was an Argentine philosopher whose career spanned the late twentieth and early twenty-first century. One of her legacies was contributing to the broader project of critiquing "white feminism"—a form of theory that ignores how factors like race or sexuality affect women differently. This is where her concept of "world-traveling" comes in. She draws on the experiences of minority women moving between worlds where they're insiders to worlds where they're outsiders. "As outsiders to the mainstream, women of color in the U.S. practice 'world'-travelling, mostly out of necessity," she says.[9] She conceives of worlds that are cultural. "A 'world' in my sense may be an actual society given its dominant culture's description and construction of life.... But a 'world' can also be such a society given a non-dominant construction."[10] For Lugones, worlds vary in size and may encompass other worlds. For instance, the "world of fashion" exists within the larger "world of US culture" or the culture of another country.

Worlds shape our sense of self. For example, a Black or Latina woman may be a particular type of person, with her distinctive way of being in the world, when she is with other Blacks or Latinas. Yet when she finds herself in the broader US world, such as a workplace where she interacts with white people, she may move her body, speak, or otherwise inhabit the world differently. Maybe her tone is more deferential than it is when she's with people of her own race. This is the idea behind the notion of "code switching," which refers to the way we change our tone or vocabulary depending on different social contexts. Lugones herself uses the example of being seen as playful in her "home world" as opposed to being perceived as serious in the white/Anglo world. She sums up her account in these words: "Those of us who are 'world'-travellers have the distinct experience of being different in different 'worlds' and of having the capacity to remember other 'worlds' and our selves in them."[11]

Sometimes we enter certain worlds out of necessity, and these are often marked by "arrogance."[12] They're hierarchical. For example, in an arrogant setting, a white person won't bother making small talk with the Black or brown cashier, when he would with someone of his own race. Or in a business setting, someone (unthinkingly or not) disregards the input of a colleague of color, all the while favoring the same idea when expressed by a white colleague. Entering such worlds involves risk. But there are worlds that we can also enter *lovingly.* Connecting with other people in worlds that we travel to lovingly allows us to "identify with them," "to understand *what it is to be them,*" and also "*what it is to be ourselves in their eyes.*"[13] Just as traveling to another country can help us better understand other people and make visible what's distinctive about our home, so too traveling between worlds helps us view ourselves and others differently. We need to embody what Lugones calls "playfulness" to see people in new and loving ways: "The playful attitude involves openness to surprise, openness to being a fool, openness to self-construction or reconstruction."[14] Instead of imposing our view on others, we allow ourselves to be flexible and open to change. According to her, a playful attitude allows women of different cultures and races to relate to each other and forge "unity."[15] But this could be said of all our efforts to find common ground. Traveling between worlds can transform us—on condition that we adopt a playful attitude and shed our arrogant ways of viewing others.

How can we embody a loving gaze? How can we learn to look at others otherwise? In her 2014 article "A Phenomenology of Hesitation: Interrupting Racializing Habits of Seeing," feminist philosopher Alia Al-Saji broaches this question. She says that to look at others "otherwise," or differently, we need to learn to *feel* otherwise about them. Perceiving and emotion go hand in hand. For instance, if I've been scared after a home invasion, the same shadows in my apartment that once were unremarkable will now look threatening. According to Al-Saji, when it comes to relating to other people, to feel otherwise, there needs to be an "interruption," a way of short-circuiting our habitual ways of being with them. To achieve such interruption, we need "the creation of situations and attachments that bring hesitation about."[16] By this she means that new environments (e.g., a group of friends or a family) can interrupt our automatic emotional responses to other people. To illustrate this claim, she mentions the experience of her partner, who is not Muslim, when he became part of an extended family where some women wore veils and others did not. This setting was a new "affective environment" that interrupted his unthinking reactions to veiled women and taught him to see them otherwise. He learned that the decision to veil or not is much more complicated than non-Muslim culture suggested to him. In this sense, he learned to approach this and other questions with openness and curiosity about "interruptions" of this kind.

By changing our perceptions and feelings about others, we can also shape the way we view ourselves. The two go hand in hand. If, as thin people, we look at fat bodies with disapproval, how will we relate to our own bodies? We'll live in fear of changes in our own size and shape. And if fat people feel demonized, until they learn to see themselves differently, won't they also view their bodies with trepidation? By learning to regard ourselves and others in new ways, we can shed the limiting body shame that preys on us.

Tying these ideas together, we find that new settings, when we enter them with openness and even a sense of playfulness, can transform us at our core. Lugones goes so far as to say that we can begin "loving" each other.[17] And when we do, we can begin to remake the world. Worlds aren't static. As Lugones teaches us, playful world-traveling allows for the "reconstruction" of ourselves *and* of worlds themselves. My vision is for us to remake the world in more equitable ways. This book's goal has been to challenge diet culture, the culture that disordered eating and negative body image thrive on. How can we change this culture? How can we remake the world?

How to Remake Worlds

Thanks to Heidegger, we have a useful vocabulary for understanding how our identities alter how we approach the objects in the world.

Now let's combine this with Lugones's idea that we can be playful and creative with our identities. In other words, the people we choose to spend time with, and the sense of openness we take with us in new encounters, can shape us and our world. This allows us to see new possibilities where we previously did not. We might try to view the world as a feminist or as an environmental activist, for example, or imagine ourselves in new roles, such as parent or artist.

Yet this insight doesn't imply that we should just take on any identity we come across. We must also pause. What values are my own? Who do I want to become? This is where another Heideggerian idea comes into play. After spending much of *Being and Time* describing the structure of worlds, Heidegger explains how facing our mortality asks us to reconsider who we are. He contrasts two ways of leading our lives. First, people can live inauthentically. As we coast from friend group to friend group, we might adopt the same hobbies our friends have, we might parrot the way they speak, we might vote the way they do, and so on. People living inauthentically have not confronted the truth that their time on this planet is limited and that they may be wasting it on doing what others do. The second option is that people can live authentically. This implies pausing to reconsider how we're living, choosing values of our own, and leading our lives according to them. Without getting too deep into Heidegger, we can appreciate how the desire to live authentically requires us to look at our lives as a whole, from beginning to end.

This discussion may feel like it has taken us far afield from diet culture. But it hasn't. Heidegger's recommendations regarding authenticity put into relief something we know deep inside: Our concerns about appearance are trivial compared to other things that are important to us. I once came across an anti-diet-culture slogan: "No one is going to stand up at your funeral and say . . . 'She had a small waist and a great thigh gap.'" Of course not! I want to be remembered for my intelligence as a philosopher, my dedication to family, friends, and students, and even my playful and open willingness to have a deep relationship with my dog. And I expect similar responses from you all. You may want to be recognized for your devotion as a friend or as a parent, for your wit or your kindness, for your success in your professional life, or your zeal for an unusual hobby. I bet that none of you want your tombstone to read: "She dieted."

This is not to say that beauty is unimportant. Revering human beauty is part and parcel of cultures across history and around the globe, and this reverence will likely endure so long as we tread the earth. But is our present relationship to human beauty balanced? When the pursuit of physical ideals, such as thinness, is in conflict with other aspects of our lives—caring for our families, dedicating ourselves to callings, or honoring our own health—then something has gone awry. How much weight do we want to give to fashioning a perfect body? Do a few pounds matter all that much? In the end, as the writer Leo Tolstoy put it, all we will amount to is "stench and worms."[18] In this context, his words suggest we should be more than the playthings of the beauty industry. Instead, we have the choice to be playful, alive, and sensual, rather than locked in the mindset inherited from diet culture. These words also summon us to *create* a world where we won't feel that our sense of self and our livelihood depend on how attractive or how thin we are.

Throughout my second round of eating disorder counseling, I had to ask myself these hard questions. In September 2020, I knew my life had taken a wrong turn when I found myself incapacitated from dieting and unable to care for my dog. I realized that I needed to make peace with my body so I could devote myself to the activities and people that mattered to me. And I recognized that I could no longer divide my aims between chasing thinness and achieving goals that were authentically my own. Two years later, as the end of counseling neared, these concerns felt even more pressing. I felt confident that I had chosen the right course of action by resuming counseling, learning to eat, and challenging my limiting beliefs about my body size. Yet I still feared losing my identity as someone who was underweight and ultra skinny. I called the voices that told me to start dieting again my "Night Demons." Without them to keep me in check, who would I become?

Thinking philosophically about my life as a whole in the way I've depicted here helped me resist the Night Demons. It helped me keep the bigger picture in the forefront of my mind. My identity as a *feminist* also helped. For me, feminism has meant understanding the attitudes and social circumstances that perpetuate gender inequality. It has also required a commitment to challenging these attitudes and circumstances. When I write about feminist philosophy, I invite my readers to acknowledge the sexism that is still baked into much of what we do. Recently, a friend sent me a picture of a svelte woman on a package for a low-calorie cheese because he saw it as an illustration of how we use depictions of feminine thinness to market products. Why? In a society dominated by the thin ideal, slenderness helps us sell more goods. These are the tiny things we need to recognize if we are to remake the world. Naturally, there are other issues—the gender wage gap, discrimination, access to healthcare—that ought to be combated. Feminist philosophy has helped me grapple with problems, small and large, and it has supported my efforts to uproot my own issues with eating and body image.

My story doesn't imply that you need to adopt the label "feminist" to resist diet culture, let alone recover from disordered eating. You may have negative associations with the word, or you may not like political labels at all. This identity has helped me, but it might not serve you. This chapter is simply an invitation to scrutinize which parts of yourself are self-destructive and which are self-affirming.

Once we strive to look over the whole of our lives and live according to what we truly value and what brings us true pleasure, how do we change the world? Here are a few examples that show that it is not as hard as people often think. Simple acts of choosing what you have around you, and what you do with it, go a long way.

I opened this chapter with my experience with mirrors, and I've mentioned Renee Engeln's concerns about mirrors in gyms. For her, their presence encourages us to think of exercise as a means to sculpt our bodies, rather than an activity we can enjoy for its own sake. Of course, mirrors are useful for coordinating clothing, removing pesky stray eyelashes, and the like. Mirrors can even be used to ensure you are using the proper technique or form in some exercises. Still, I invite you to reflect on why you use mirrors and when using mirrors is to your detriment. Heidegger speaks of the "for-the-sake-of-which" of a tool. Is your mirror for the sake of body checking—a critical examination of your so-called flaws? Or does it serve another purpose? What is the identity—dieter, fashionista, or something else—that informs your use of mirrors?

Many of us also weigh ourselves compulsively—sometimes several times a day. In my adult life, I've owned six scales. I've always ended up discarding them (I even took a hammer to one!) because I realized they were a tool for surveilling myself. My weight always went down once I acquired a scale, and in my better moments, I recognized that I was on a slippery slope to damaging eating habits. So, out the scale went, each time. Perhaps you identify with this worry. Or perhaps scales are useful to you. You may be monitoring your weight out of a health concern or because you're trying to build muscle as part of a weightlifting regimen. Again, I don't mean to dictate a one-size-fits-all prescription but to recommend asking: Where does the need to have a scale flow from?

The same goes for food. Is food merely fuel to you? In what contexts is it sustenance or something else? On most days, food might be fuel—just a tool to keep your body functioning. On other days, however, it might have a cultural significance. Think of the abundant meals of those who celebrate Thanksgiving. Is food a means to express yourself? Do you enjoy cooking tasty meals? In that case, food choices might spring from a sense of creativity, instead of functionality. Again, this might depend on circumstances. On school mornings, I cook simple eggs because they keep my hunger satisfied during long teaching hours. But on other occasions, such as my virtual cooking lessons, creating a delicious meal is a gratifying challenge, and regardless of how it turns out, the activity strengthens my bond with my mother.

Similar considerations apply to restricting our food intake or eliminating food groups. Do you fast to alter your metabolism? Or for religious reasons? Are you a vegetarian or vegan out of ethical concerns? Or because you believe that this diet can enhance your athletic performance? And more to this book's topic, let's pause to consider the food choices that come with disordered eating. Does restricting food stem from a sense that eating less equals greater self-worth? Do you derive a feeling of superiority from controlling your appetite? Do you believe that you're vanquishing something "awesome" through starvation? In chapter 6, when we considered eating disorders during the pandemic, we learned that restriction could provide a sense of the sublime. Most of my life, restriction meant security. I could shield myself from the judgment of others. When modeling was on my mind, it also meant beauty: "Nothing tastes better than skinny feels." When I was overwhelmed by the pandemic, it meant control. I couldn't end the pandemic, but I could avoid eating. Again, to develop more resilience against the onslaught of skinny, we should question how our sense of self affects our food choices.

So far I've discussed things—ordinary objects like mirrors and scales—and items like food, which you might not at first conceive of as things. They're part of our physical environment. But what about representations in art? What can paintings, photographs, sculptures, or movies teach us about remaking the world? And what lessons can we take from everyday media, such as the images of Instagram or videos of TikTok?

Regarding art, feminist philosopher A. W. Eaton appeals to Aristotle's notion of habituation to describe how we can reform our "tastes" in bodies.[19] For instance, Aristotle did not think that we're born courageous or temperate. Rather, because we have a baseline capacity to feel feelings of fear and confidence or pleasure and pain, we can train ourselves to develop these virtues of character. So too with our tastes in artistic representation. We can train ourselves to "enjoy and hate finely."[20] Rational argument can do little to dislodge these tastes. Delightful, enticing, or fanciful images, however, can challenge our love of and disgust with different physiques. As an example, Eaton cites contemporary high art such as Leonard Nimoy's "The Full Body

Project," which pushes us to look at fat persons differently. His photos include "high-contrast black-and-white photographs of unclothed fat women who often strike classical poses informed by art masterpieces such as Marcel Duchamp's *Nude Descending a Staircase.*"[21] But Eaton also mentions pop stars such as Missy Elliot and Meghan Trainor, whose song "All About That Bass" "sparked something of a national conversation about fat positivity."[22] While Eaton has fat bodies in mind, we can broaden her argument to other bodies historically cast as unattractive (e.g., Black bodies). Art can teach us to view ourselves and others in more fair-minded and imaginative ways.

On the topic of everyday representations, the conversation is complicated. As mentioned in chapter 9, some psychological studies have suggested that media literacy has more limited effects than we might hope. For example, warning labels about modified images can cause us to focus on our bodies rather than reconsider the images themselves, and may even make us feel worse.[23] This finding reminds us that reason alone may not serve us in reenvisioning the world more equitably. Telling ourselves that an image is unrealistic isn't enough to stop being swayed by it. Nonetheless, we can borrow a lesson from Eaton's discussion—namely, that the more tasteful our representations of diverse bodies become, the more we can learn to see others otherwise. Whether it's high art or our social media feeds, let's consciously consider what we consume.

The questions I've raised in this section call on us to fashion our physical worlds and media landscapes in ways that empower us. Let's also note that such changes are never done in a vacuum. The existentialist thinker Jean-Paul Sartre invites us to consider the effects of our actions on others. In his famous 1945 lecture "Existentialism Is a Humanism," he says, "I am responsible for myself and for everyone else. I am creating a certain image of man of my own choosing. In choosing myself, I choose man."[24] As hyperbolic as his words might sound, Sartre is pointing to an important truth: We don't make choices in a bubble. When we restrict food at a meal with others, when we post videos under #SkinnyTok, or when we praise an acquaintance for their weight loss without knowing its causes, we're enshrining thinness as a beauty standard. Conversely, when we help someone in eating-disorder recovery shop for groceries, when we mute social media that focuses on dieting, or when we listen to others' body image concerns with an open mind, then we're combating this standard. As we've seen, communities of resistance serve to challenge the norms and break the rules. In turn, such resistance lends us the strength to remake our worlds.

In this discussion, I've combined two ways of thinking to answer the question of how we can make our world. The first one, based on Heidegger's work, is that our identities inform how we interact with our environment, whether it's in the form of everyday objects, food, art, or social media. The second one, grounded in Lugones's work, is that we can remake ourselves through world-traveling. When we learn to perceive others otherwise, we can forge loving relationships with them and understand ourselves in new ways. In turn, when we understand ourselves in new ways, we can change the world. Reentering eating disorder counseling and being in dialogue with my counselor created a space where I could envision new possibilities for myself. One of these possibilities was to leave behind the world of food restriction. This new world was one where eating became either neutral or positive, where cooking promised creativity and connection, and where scales and mirrors no longer belonged.

What About the Natural World?

We've examined worlds through the lens of culture. But where does the natural world fit into the picture? Can it teach us anything about revolutionizing our understanding of our body and those of others?

In his book *Ecce Homo*, the nineteenth-century philosopher Friedrich Nietzsche declared, "Do not believe any idea that was not conceived while moving around outside."[25] Nietzsche, who endured debilitating migraines and stomach issues for most of his life, spent much of his philosophical career writing about the meaning of suffering.

He criticized the hope for an afterlife that would redeem our earthly sufferings. For him, this was a poisonous idea that undermined our lives. The outdoors provided a setting for him to exercise and heal from his physical illnesses. At first glance, Nietzsche's sentence merely seems to confirm conventional wisdom. We go for a walk to "clear our minds." Or we have a "shower thought" when we wash ourselves. But if we reflect on the context where he formulated his philosophy, we see that there's more to his pronouncement. Much of his walking unfolded in the Alps—mountains of dizzying heights and breathtaking views. When Nietzsche hiked, he was in *awe*.

Awe is a feeling that has attracted much attention in science and philosophy in recent years. In psychology, Dacher Keltner, a leading figure in studies of emotion, probes the meaning of this experience. In his book *Awe*, he defines it as the feeling awakened "in the presence of something vast that transcends your current understanding of the world."[26] We can experience this emotion when faced with events of great moral significance, works of art, and in nature. In his discussion of "wild awe," Keltner points to the health benefits of practices like forest bathing, "where people are led through immersive awe experience in forests—for example, walking, taking in scents, feeling leaves and bark on the skin and with the hands, contemplating for a moment a tree and its remarkable designs."[27] These practices can help reduce the likelihood of conditions such as cardiovascular disease, diabetes, depression, anxiety, and cancer.[28] More to our point, Keltner wonders whether "wild awe" can give us a clearer perspective on our lives and surrounding world. He thinks so. Awe challenges a "mean egotism" that makes us narcissistic and partisan.[29]

Contemporary research in philosophy also explores how awe affects our understanding of ourselves and of the world. In *Wonderstruck*, Helen De Cruz conceives of awe as an "emotion we sense when we perceive or conceptualize vastness, combined with a need for cognitive accommodation"—that is, "we want to make space in our minds for this vast thing."[30] Looking up at a starry sky from a mountaintop can elicit such a feeling. Closely related to awe is wonder, the "emotion that arises from a glimpse at the unknown terrain which lies just beyond the fringes of our current understanding."[31] For De Cruz, wonder doesn't require vastness; it can come from things like looking at an insect under a microscope or finding an interesting fossil. Both awe and wonder are "epistemic notions," that is, they motivate us to learn more about our surroundings. Crucially, they're "self-transcendent emotions"—they compel us to overcome a myopic focus on ourselves.[32]

Based on these ideas, let's ask: Could being in nature help us reconsider our perspective on our body? Could it even lead to improved body image? The data is relatively limited, but research in psychology has examined this possibility. For example, a 2018 study published in *Body Image* offered evidence in favor of this connection. The study combined experiments where test subjects viewed images of either natural or built environments, went on a walk in a natural or built environment, or explored a designed green space. The authors reported that their results corroborated previous work "indicating that self-reported exposure to nature was significantly associated with more positive body appreciation."[33] A 2024 review of literature on body image and nature observed that "there is now a broad base of evidence showing that nature exposure is reliably associated with body image outcomes."[34] But it also noted the limitations of these studies; some factors, such as geographical focus, haven't yet been researched sufficiently. It concluded that "nevertheless, there are good reasons to think that nature exposure can be leveraged to support healthier body image outcomes for individuals, communities, and populations."[35] Based on this review and related work, I'm hopeful that psychology will confirm the intuition that immersing ourselves in nature can offer one more way, besides those I already discussed, for us to be in our bodies, and to provide endless new opportunities for curiosity and worldmaking.

As a final note, I want to mention that for those times when we cannot get out into nature right now, there are other ways to find awe in nature. One way is to seek out and take pleasure in artists who explore the body-world connection in their work. For example, Elsa Marie Keefe's series of self-portraits in nature explores how the natural world can heal our relationship with our bodies. In the artist's words: "We are all born wild, and being naked is our primal truth. My photographic practice is about remembering our sacred nature and celebrating how our bodies mirror and embody the natural world."[36] Keefe's art combines the idea that art can alter our tastes in bodies and the suggestion that our connection to the natural world transforms us for the better.

Nietzsche's pronouncement on only believing ideas conceived outdoors isn't about remaking the natural world, but about how the natural world can remake us. When we're in awe, we're taken away from everyday concerns and come back to our lives with a renewed sense of curiosity or purpose. In turn, we can draw on such inspiration to remake our cultural worlds.

Since I reentered eating disorder counseling, Carol and I have walked the forty minutes between our home and the doggy beach off Key Biscayne every few weeks. I've always daydreamed as we cover the path to this beach, sometimes about my philosophical writing, sometimes about my life. In November 2022, Dalit and I agreed that if I do not have any lapses, I can conclude eating disorder counseling after the end-of-year holidays. In the past two and a half years of counseling, I've wondered what a life free of disordered eating would look like. This possibility frightens me because I worry about the judgment of others about my body. But it also inspires me because I never want to find myself dizzy with hunger and unable to care for Carol.

On December 7, several weeks after that conversation, Carol and I make our way to the beach. By 8:30, the sun has risen, and she is panting. I'm hot, too, and slip off my sneakers. With her in my arms, I wade in as cool waves lap back and forth. I scan the water: The sunlight has carved a glittering path from my feet all the way to the cotton clouds gathering at the horizon. No matter how many times I view them, Miami's sunrises always fill me with awe. In that moment, I feel free—free from worries about my diet, my body, and my future. That bright morning blesses me.

Epilogue

January 2023. Over two years have elapsed since the night my world collapsed. Monday, the 9th, will be my final session with Dalit. The end of eating disorder counseling. And with it, the end of my eating disorder? I wonder. From time to time, I still feel oppressed by that tyrant: Thinness. I avoid restricting, but the thought that I've committed a crime by gaining a little over ten pounds burdens me. My efforts are imperfect. Just a week ago, I struggled to sleep because I was hungry. But I rose from bed to have some banana bread instead of trying to power through my pangs of hunger. I knew there should be no guilt, but my Night Demons lingered.

This week, I'm mulling over options for my concluding recipe. I plan on cooking on Saturday as I'll be speaking with Dalit in the afternoon, and my Sundays are always busy with a Zoom of other sorts: happy hour with my mother and sister.

In fall 2022, Dalit mentioned trying new recipes. I made a promise to myself then: As daunting as it sounded, I would give sushi a shot. A new Japanese restaurant and sushi ingredient place had opened a ten-minute walk from me. It would be the perfect challenge. But I let the idea slide as school caught up with me. Instead, I continued learning new recipes thanks to my mother, who dislikes sushi.

On Thursday, January 5, I remember my old resolution. Sushi it will be. I need to end with a flourish!

I scour recipes online and watch several YouTube tutorials about how to make rolls. Crafts are not my strong suit, and this resembles craftwork more than cooking. Am I up to the challenge? But what else can I make that would be as symbolic a victory as creating sushi? I have learned to cook pasta Bolognese, Chinese chicken, chicken Marengo, eggplant parmigiana, beef bourguignon, Moroccan tagine, and so many more recipes. I will teach myself how to make sushi. Even if I have to do it alone. Even if I make a mess of it.

On Amazon I order a sushi-making kit, which comes with rolling mats, chopsticks, a paddle, and a spreader for the rice. That's easy enough. The only part I am worried about is collecting the ingredients. Will I look like a novice in the sushi supply shop? When I arrive at the store a couple of days later, I feel embarrassed as I stare at the array of ingredients, unsure where to start in my attempt to choose the right rice and nori. But one of the attendants notices me in my confusion. He is friendly, and I succeed in acquiring the requisite ingredients. I purchase the carrots, salmon, cucumber, and avocado from Whole Foods.

Saturday night comes around. I pull on my yellow apron, a Christmas gift from my sister. In the past year, I have been showered with cooking-related gifts: a beautiful wooden spoon and spatula set from a close friend, an uncountable number of devices from my mother and sister—a massive pot for stews, a high-powered blender to replace my tiny Nutribullet, a grater, tongs, and so on.

I lay my ingredients out. I know how important mise-en-place is by now. Gone are the days of catching up with my mother and measuring ingredients as I go along. I pour the rice into a pot with some water. Once it's on the stove, I check the side of the bag to see how long it needs to cook. Forty-five minutes. Far longer than the twenty minutes I'm accustomed to when preparing regular white rice. But as my godmother Chris always says, c'est la vie. At the very least, the lengthy wait will give me enough time to peel the cucumber and avocado and to sear the salmon. What about the carrots? I should save them for another time. Maybe for a pasta Bolognese. Isn't it wise to keep things simple as a beginner? The rice is still cooking, so I reacquaint myself with putting the rolls together. I pour myself a glass of wine and open YouTube up. The rolls look perfect, and the chef makes the technique seem easy. Yet the doubt I experienced on Thursday creeps in. Will I flub the whole thing?

I'm very hungry by the time the rice is ready, and I rush the cooling segment so that I can eat dinner before midnight. I feel the gnawing hunger I used to experience when I denied myself food. But I haven't restricted. It's just the hunger I have, a part of being human. It has taken me two years to learn to accept my hunger and not to fight it.

The rice is now cool enough. I place the nori on the mat. Then I spread the rice evenly across its surface. Should I start with a cucumber roll? Won't that be the easiest? At least I won't be working with multiple ingredients. I roll it. To my surprise, it looks decent enough: the rice has stayed within the edges of the nori, and it appears I have used the right amount. The roll looks like a roll! After that, I chop it into bite-sized pieces. Alas, the pieces look a bit uneven, and the cucumber is threatening to slip out of a couple of them. I smile, both amused at the sloppiness and proud that it isn't worse. I take a few photos of my first quasi-successful attempt at making a sushi roll. Given the shape of my cucumber roll, I abandon the idea of assembling the cucumber and avocado in one roll. Onto the avocado solo. And then onto the salmon roll. Again, I'm met with surprise when I finish cutting them. Behold semi-neat sushi!

Perhaps the YouTube videos have paid off. Perhaps all my virtual cooking lessons have also given me some facility in the kitchen. And perhaps, too, it's the desire to perfect my final meal for Dalit. I place the three rolls on my plate and pour soy sauce into a tiny espresso cup. I take them to my desk and snap a picture of them. Borrowing from my favorite Fatboy Slim lyrics of the '90s, I think to myself, You've come a long way, baby.

These are the photos I share with Dalit on Monday. Was the sushi good? Good, but not restaurant good. Acceptable. I smile as I recount the experience of making it. I also show her the dumplings I cooked with my mother and sister for New Year's Eve and the cinnamon buns we baked the next day. I'm proud of myself. But I also am starting to feel the pain of our goodbye. My throat tightens as I continue with my tales of holiday cooking. I pause, out of material. Dalit interjects. "Let's talk about this session, our last hour of counseling." My eyes well up, and I start to say something. But nothing comes out. I've anticipated crying. I know from years of therapy that there's no avoiding tears during a final session. I sobbed during my last one in graduate school with a therapist I had seen for nine years. And I wept in 2019, when I concluded therapy with someone whom I had only seen for a year but had quickly grown attached to. Given my history with Dalit, it's hard not to cry in these final minutes.

We speak a bit during that time—not of my journey to get to this moment, but of what's to come: I'm dating someone new, I'm soon giving several talks, and I'm working on a book. "I feel goose bumps as you speak," Dalit says. She has never said anything so personal. Her words move me. But wracked with sobs, I have none of my own. She sits with me as I cry. And as with other final therapy sessions, we wrap up early. There is nothing to plan for, no "next time we meet" to discuss. I smile through tears as I say goodbye and leave the Zoom meeting. That's it. My eyes dry up, minute by minute. I've reached the end. The end of eating disorder counseling.

I FIRST DRAFTED THESE WORDS on November 20, 2023—my thirty-eighth birthday. Since then, I've had nearly two years to ponder my life and the philosophy I've crafted from it. I first developed my ideas about bodily alienation as I began to think about thinspo while writing my dissertation. Alongside, my own sense of estrangement from my body seesawed. During graduate school and my early years as a philosophy professor, learning about the feminist ideas presented in this book—those of Simone de Beauvoir and Nancy Bauer, of Sandra Bartky and Susan Bordo, of Audre Lorde and María Lugones—pushed me toward healthier heights. But the force of diet culture and the beauty industry pulled me down. Down my portions would go, down my weight would go. Until I could go no further.

My second round of eating disorder counseling propelled me. Yet to say that I have reached "escape velocity" would be an overstatement. I envy anyone who no longer feels burdened by the norm of feminine thinness. I have gone through days when restriction seemed more sensible than cooking. I have lost some of the weight I gained during counseling. But I've also gained it back. Rarely has a week gone by without any banana bread baking. And rarely have any days of dieting lasted any longer. Homemade meals taste better than skinny feels.

Writing this book has also driven me. Like Simone de Beauvoir, who for a long time hesitated "before writing a book on woman," I have wavered about composing a book that would meld my personal experience with disordered eating and my philosophical training. According to Beauvoir, "Enough ink has flowed over the quarrel about feminism; it is now almost over."[1] So too, it would seem, with the slenderness standard. Still, Beauvoir noted that at a time when women's social position was in flux, with women gaining the vote and other rights across the world, feminism was still subject to debate. Similarly, in 2025, as I conclude this book, much has been written about thinness. Yet the progressions and regressions in our beauty standards still demand scrutiny. Why does dieting to fit into a size 2 or 4 continue to feel compelling? Why has heroin chic morphed into thinspo, and thinspo into #SkinnyTok?

If thin is still in, then there's a place for this book. By looking at this fetish through a philosophical lens, I hope to have helped readers see through its falsity. Worshipping thinness is idolatry. It's a religion that has been peddled for centuries, at times as a replacement for traditional faith, at others as part of its substance. In contrast, if we reconnect with our bodies, as I've counseled in these pages, perhaps we can save ourselves from this idol. You might not go so far as embracing Tantra—I'm not sure if I've yet reached that point, as compelling as I find Lama Yeshe's portrayal of the tradition. Still, as you close this book, I hope you can find healing through self-care—by practicing intuitive eating or intuitive exercise, by savoring the body's pleasures or enjoying the world around you—and that you share this message with others. Self-care and community care go together.

Not every reader will have shared my history. Perhaps you've never suffered from a diagnosable eating disorder. Perhaps your experiences were more dire than mine. Perhaps your struggles took other forms:

bulimia or binge-eating, for instance. Or perhaps you chased different false pleasures, different idols, and see your journey overlapping with mine. However you came to this book, I hope you leave it with ideas and tools that will always be with you, so that *we* can face the tyranny of thinness in solidarity. We can do this by listening to each other. I've woven my story through the ideas of our feminist foremothers. Now I want to hear yours. As Audre Lorde so wisely put it, "I am not free while any woman is unfree, even when her shackles are very different from my own."[2]

Notes

Introduction

1 See Kim Chernin, *The Obsession: Reflections on the Tyranny of Slenderness* (Harper & Row, 1981).
2 Jennifer Thomas and Jenni Schaefer, *Almost Anorexic: Is My (or My Loved One's) Relationship with Food a Problem?* (Hazelden, 2013).
3 Audre Lorde, *A Burst of Light and Other Essays* (Ixia, 2017), 130.

Chapter 1. Lessons Learned and Unlearned

1 Sarah Grogan, *Body Image: Understanding Body Dissatisfaction in Men, Women and Children*, 4th ed. (Routledge, 2022), 163.
2 Grogan, *Body Image*, 163–64.
3 Grogan, 4.
4 Grogan, 4.
5 Grogan, 51.
6 Sabrina Strings elaborates on these limitations in her journal article "How the Use of BMI Fetishizes White Embodiment and Racializes Fat Phobia," *AMA Journal of Ethics* 25, no. 7 (2023): E535–39, https://doi.org/10.1001/amajethics.2023.535 (accessed September 11, 2025).
7 World Health Organization, "Moderate and Severe Thinness, Underweight, Overweight, Obesity," n.d., https://apps.who.int/nutrition/landscape/help.aspx?menu=0&helpid=420 (accessed September 11, 2025).
8 Hilary E. A. Whyte, S. M. Findlay, and Canadian Paediatric Society, Adolescent Health Committee, "Dieting in Adolescence," *Paediatrics & Child Health* 9, no. 7 (2004): 487–91, https://doi.org/10.1093/pch/9.7.487 (accessed September 12, 2025).
9 Ioanna Kontele et al., "Parental Dieting and Correlation with Disordered Eating Behaviours in Adolescents: A Narrative Review," *Adolescents* 3, no. 3 (2023): 538–49, https://doi.org/10.3390/adolescents3030038.

10 Dianne Neumark-Sztainer et al., "Eating, Activity, and Weight-Related Problems from Adolescence to Adulthood," *American Journal of Preventive Medicine* 55, no. 2 (2018): 133–41, https://doi.org/10.1016/j.amepre.2018.04.032.

11 Kirrilly M. Pursey et al., "Disordered Eating, Body Image Concerns, and Weight Control Behaviors in Primary School Aged Children: A Systematic Review and Meta-analysis of Universal–Selective Prevention Interventions," *International Journal of Eating Disorders* 54, no. 10 (2021): 1730–65, https://doi.org/10.1002/eat.23571.

12 Pursey et al., "Disordered Eating, Body Image Concerns."

13 See Maja Batista et al., "Predictors of Eating Disorder Risk in Anorexia Nervosa Adolescents," *Acta Clinica Croatica* 57, no. 3 (2018): 399–410, https://doi.org/10.20471/acc.2018.57.03.01.

14 Marya Hornbacher, *Wasted: A Memoir of Anorexia and Bulimia* (HarperCollins, 1998), 6.

15 Hornbacher, *Wasted*, 6.

16 See Sarah Barakat et al. "Risk Factors for Eating Disorders: Findings from a Rapid Review," *Journal of Eating Disorders* 11, no. 8 (2023): 1–31, https://doi.org/10.1186/s40337-022-00717-4.

17 See Sasha Gorrell and Stuart B. Murray, "Eating Disorders in Males," *Child and Adolescent Psychiatric Clinics of North America* 28, no. 4 (2019): 641–51.

18 National Association of Anorexia Nervosa and Associated Disorders (ANAD), "Eating Disorder Statistics." https://anad.org/eating-disorder-statistic (accessed August 1, 2025).

19 ANAD, "Eating Disorder Statistics."

20 ANAD, "Eating Disorder Statistics."

21 Nadia Micali et al., "Lifetime and 12-Month Prevalence of Eating Disorders Amongst Women in Mid-Life: A Population-Based Study of Diagnoses and Risk Factors," *BMC Medicine* 15, no. 12 (2017), https://doi.org/10.1186/s12916-016-0766-4.

22 Pierre Bourdieu, *Distinction: A Social Critique of the Judgement of Taste*, trans. Richard Nice (Harvard University Press, 1984), 6.

23 Sabrina Strings, *Fearing the Black Body: The Racial Origins of Fat Phobia* (New York University Press, 2019), 6.

24 Strings, *Fearing the Black Body*, 63.
25 Strings, *Fearing the Black Body*, 91.
26 Quoted in Elizabeth Wissinger, *This Year's Model: Fashion, Media, and the Making of Glamour* (New York University Press, 2015), 124.
27 Kate Manne, *Unshrinking: How to Face Fatphobia* (Crown, 2024), 50.
28 Manne, *Unshrinking*, 49.
29 Luna Dolezal, *The Body and Shame: Feminism, Phenomenology, and the Socially Shaped Body* (Lexington, 2015), xv.
30 Corydon Ireland, "Fijian Girls Succumb to Western Dysmorphia," *Harvard Gazette*, March 19, 2009, https://news.harvard.edu/gazette/story/2009/03/fijian-girls-succumb-to-western-dysmorphia (accessed September 13, 2025).
31 For an extensive discussion of men's body image, I recommend chapter 4 ("Men and Body Image") of Grogan's *Body Image*.
32 Naomi Wolf, *The Beauty Myth: How Images of Beauty Are Used Against Women* (HarperPerennial, 2002), 10–11.
33 Susan Bordo, *Unbearable Weight: Feminism, Western Culture, and the Body* (University of California Press, 1993), 155.
34 Bordo, *Unbearable Weight*, 155.
35 Elizabeth Patton, "Why Did Ultrathin Models Make a Comeback at Fashion Week?" *New York Times*, March 11, 2023, https://www.nytimes.com/2023/03/11/fashion/why-did-ultrathin-models-make-a-comeback-at-fashion-week.html.
36 See Renee Engeln, *Beauty Sick: How the Cultural Obsession with Appearance Hurts Girls and Women* (HarperCollins, 2017), 241; see chapter 11 ("Turning Down the Volume") for an explanation of our evolutionary preferences.
37 See Heather Widdows's explanation of work on evolutionary preferences in *Perfect Me: Beauty as an Ethical Ideal* (Princeton University Press, 2018).
38 Widdows, *Perfect Me*, 21.
39 Édith Breton et al., "Developmental Trajectories of Eating Disorder Symptoms: A Longitudinal Study from Early Adolescence to Young Adulthood." *Journal of Eating Disorders* 10, no. 1 (2022), https://doi.org/10.1186/s40337-022-00603-z.

Chapter 2. Girlhood, or the Shock of Seeing Yourself Seen

1 Aron is quoted in Sarah Bakewell, *At the Existentialist Café: Freedom, Being, and Apricot Cocktails* (Other Press, 2016), 3.

2 Simone de Beauvoir, *The Second Sex*, (Vintage Books, 2011), 283.

3 Rae Langton, *Sexual Solipsism: Philosophical Essays on Pornography and Objectification* (Oxford University Press, 2009), 228–29.

4 See Laura Mulvey, "Visual Pleasure and Narrative Cinema," *Screen* 16, no. 3 (1975): 6–18, https://doi.org/10.1093/screen/16.3.6.

5 Martha Nussbaum, "Objectification," *Philosophy and Public Affairs* 24, no. 4 (1995): 249–91.

6 See Nancy Bauer, "Simone de Beauvoir on the Allure of Self-Objectification," in *Feminist Metaphysics: Explorations in the Ontology of Sex, Gender and the Self*, ed. Charlotte Witt (Springer, 2011).

7 Renee Engeln, *Beauty Sick: How the Cultural Obsession with Appearance Hurts Girls and Women* (HarperCollins, 2017), 47.

8 Kristin Zeiler, "A Phenomenology of Excorporation, Bodily Alienation, and Resistance: Rethinking Sexed and Racialized Embodiment," *Hypatia* 28, no. 1 (2013), 80.

9 Engeln, *Beauty Sick*, 65.

10 Engeln, *Beauty Sick*, 84, 79.

11 Aristotle, *Nicomachean Ethics*, trans. W. D. Ross, http://classics.mit.edu/Aristotle/nicomachaen.4.iv.html (accessed October 6, 2025).

12 Luna Dolezal, *The Body and Shame: Feminism, Phenomenology, and the Socially Shaped Body* (Lexington, 2015), 3.

13 Dolezal, *Body and Shame*, 5.

14 Dolezal, *Body and Shame*, xv.

15 Beauvoir, *Second Sex*, 321.

16 See Iris Marion Young, "Menstrual Meditations," in *On Female Body Experience: "Throwing Like a Girl" and Other Essays* (Oxford University Press, 2005).

17 Engeln, *Beauty Sick*, 91.

18 See Sandra Bartky, "Foucault, Femininity, and the Modernization of Patriarchal Power," in *Femininity and Domination: Studies in the Phenomenology of Oppression* (Routledge, 1990).

19 Heather Widdows, *Perfect Me: Beauty as an Ethical Ideal* (Princeton University Press, 2018), 161.

20 Widdows, *Perfect Me*, 174.

21 See Nancy Bauer's chapter "What Philosophy Can't Teach Us About Sexual Objectification" in *How to Do Things with Pornography* (Harvard University Press, 2015).

22 See chapter 12 of Engeln's *Beauty Sick*, "Stop the Body Talk."

23 Jaclyn A. Siegel, Virginia Ramseyer Winter, Mackenzie Cook, "'It Really Presents a Struggle for Females, Especially My Little Girl': Exploring Fathers' Experiences Discussing Body Image with Their Young Daughters," *Body Image* 36 (2021): 84–94, https://doi.org/10.1016/j.bodyim.2020.11.001.

24 Engeln, *Beauty Sick*, 148.

25 Engeln, *Beauty Sick*, 148.

26 Michelle Faverio and Olivia Sidoti, "Teens, Social Media and AI Chatbots 2025," Pew Research Center, December 9, 2025, www.pewresearch.org/internet/2025/12/09/teens-social-media-and-ai-chatbots-2025.

27 Engeln, *Beauty Sick*, 175.

28 Grogan, *Body Image*, 129. Grogan relies on research published in 2013 and 2014 by Marika Tiggermann and Amy Slater.

29 Ioanna Kontele et al., "Parental Dieting and Correlation with Disordered Eating Behaviours in Adolescents: A Narrative Review," *Adolescents* 3, no. 3 (2023): 538–49, https://doi.org/10.3390/adolescents3030038.

30 Kontele, "Parental Dieting."

31 K. Jean Forney, Teresa Schwendler, Rose Marie Ward, "Examining Similarities in Eating Pathology, Negative Affect, and Perfectionism Among Peers: A Social Network Analysis," *Appetite* (2019): 236–43, https://doi.org/10.1016/j.appet.2019.03.013.

32 See Sarah Kendal, Sue Kirk, Rebecca Elvey, Roger Catchpole, and Steven Pryjmachuk, "How a Moderated Online Discussion Forum Facilitates Support for Young People with Eating Disorders," *Health Expectations* 20 (2016): 98–111, https://doi.org/10.1111/hex.12439.

33 Annelies van Eeden, Daphne van Hoeken, and Hans Hoek, "Incidence, Prevalence and Mortality of Anorexia Nervosa and Bulimia Nervosa," *Current Opinion in Psychiatry* 34, no. 6 (2021): 515–24, https://doi.org/10.1097/YCO.0000000000000739.

34 Emily M. Pisetsky et al., "Suicide attempts in women with eating disorders," *Journal of Abnormal Psychology* 122, no. 4 (2013): 1042–56, https://doi.org/10.1037/a0034902.

Chapter 3. Double Aims, Divided Aims: The Pleasures and Pains of Beauty Culture

1 Heather Widdows, *Perfect Me: Beauty as an Ethical Ideal* (Princeton University Press, 2018), 28.

2 Heather Spencer-Oatey, *Culturally Speaking. Culture, Communication and Politeness Theory*, 2nd ed. (Continuum, 2008), 3.

3 See Judith Butler, *Gender Trouble: Feminism and the Subversion of Identity* (Routledge, 1990).

4 Nancy Etcoff, *Survival of the Prettiest: The Science of Beauty* (Anchor, 1999), 39.

5 Kate Manne, *Unshrinking: How to Face Fatphobia* (Crown, 2024), 20.

6 Renee Engeln, *Beauty Sick: How the Cultural Obsession with Appearance Hurts Girls and Women* (HarperCollins, 2017), 143.

7 Engeln, *Beauty Sick*, 132.

8 Gabrielle Olya, "How Much Gen Z, Millennial, Gen X and Boomer Women Really Spend on Beauty," GoBankingRates, September 19, 2024, https://www.gobankingrates.com/saving-money/shopping/how-much-gen-z-millennial-gen-x-and-boomer-women-spend-on-beauty.

9 Future Market Insights, "Hair Straightener Market," https://www.futuremarketinsights.com/reports/hair-straightener-market (accessed October 8, 2025). Another firm's article on the topic supports this estimate: It valued the hair straightener market at $6.37 billion in 2023. See Global Market Insights, "Hair Straightener Market Size," https://www.gminsights.com/industry-analysis/hair-straightener-market (accessed October 7, 2025).

10 See Phoebe Baker Hyde, *The Beauty Experiment* (Da Capo, 2013).

11 Marilyn Frye, *The Politics of Reality: Essays in Feminist Theory* (Crossing, 1983), 2.

12 Frye, *Politics of Reality.*

13 Simone de Beauvoir, *The Second Sex*, trans. Constance Borde and Sheila Malovany-Chevallier (Vintage, 2011), 738.

14 Sandra Bartky, "Narcissism, Femininity and Alienation," *Social Theory and Practice* 8, no. 2 (1982), 127.

15 Pierre Bourdieu and Loïc Wacquant, *An Invitation to Reflexive Sociology* (University of Chicago Press, 1992), 168.

16 Cecilie Basberg Neumann, "A Dangerous Subject: The Fashion Model and the Beauty/Narcissism Double Bind," *Hypatia* 32, no. 2 (2017), 392.
17 Basberg Neumann, "Dangerous Subject," 393.
18 Nancy Bauer, "Simone de Beauvoir on the Allure of Self-Objectification," in *Feminist Metaphysics: Explorations in the Ontology of Sex, Gender and the Self*, ed. Charlotte Witt (Springer, 2011), 124.
19 Nancy Bauer, "Lady Power," *New York Times*, June 20, 2010, https://archive.nytimes.com/opinionator.blogs.nytimes.com/2010/06/20/lady-power.
20 See Iris Marion Young, "Women Recovering Our Clothes," in *On Female Body Experience: "Throwing Like a Girl" and Other Essays* (Oxford University Press, 2005).
21 See Ann J. Cahill, "Feminist Pleasure and Feminine Beautification," *Hypatia* 18, no. 4 (2003), 42–64.
22 Cahill, "Feminist Pleasure and Feminine Beautification," 61.
23 These are the words of Alysse Dalessandro quoted in Cheryl Frazier, "Beauty Labor as a Tool to Resist Antifatness," *Hypatia* 38, no. 2 (2023), 231–50, https://doi.org/10.1017/hyp.2023.22.
24 Frazier, "Beauty Labor as a Tool," 231.
25 See Chloe W. Shakin's reporting on Sanders in "Chin Hair, Laundry, Your Opinion: Women in Menopause Don't Care," *New York Times*, June 24, 2025, https://www.nytimes.com/2025/06/24/well/menopause-melani-sanders-club.html (accessed July 25, 2025).

Chapter 4. The More Things Change, the More They Remain the Same

1 Sandra Bartky, "Narcissism, Femininity and Alienation," *Social Theory and Practice* 8, no. 2 (1982), 135.
2 Bartky, "Narcissism, Femininity and Alienation," 135.
3 Bartky, "Narcissism, Femininity and Alienation," 140.
4 Timothy Hickman, "Heroin Chic: The Visual Culture of Narcotic Addiction," *Third Text* 16, no. 2 (2002), 119, https://doi.org/10.1080/09528820210138272.
5 Hickman, "Heroin Chic," 136.

6 Mary Rizzo, "Embodying Withdrawal: Abjection and the Popularity of Heroin Chic," *Michigan Feminist Studies* 15 (2001), http://hdl.handle.net/2027/spo.ark5583.0015.004.
7 Hickman, "Heroin Chic," 135.
8 See Renee Engeln, *Beauty Sick: How the Cultural Obsession with Appearance Hurts Girls and Women* (HarperCollins, 2017), 157.
9 Céline Leboeuf, "Anatomy of the Thigh Gap," *Feminist Philosophy Quarterly* 5, no. 1 (2019), 8, https://doi.org/10.5206/fpq/2019.1.7312.
10 Leboeuf, "Anatomy of the Thigh Gap," 8.
11 Leboeuf, "Anatomy of the Thigh Gap," 8.
12 Gavin Scheldrup, "The Ozempic Era," Medical University of South Carolina, August 29, 2024, https://gradstudies.musc.edu/about/blog/2024/08/the-ozempic-era.
13 For statistics on Instagram's and TikTok's reach, see Statista's article "Most Popular Social Networks Worldwide as of February 2025, by Number of Monthly Active Users," https://www.statista.com/statistics/272014/global-social-networks-ranked-by-number-of-users (accessed August 26, 2025).
14 A *New York Times* opinion piece based on interviews with Meher Ahmad and Jessica Grose and produced by Derek Arthur documents these trends. See "Why the Right Is Obsessed With Thinness: When Diet Culture Meets Conservative Morality," *New York Times*, July 30, 2025, https://www.nytimes.com/2025/07/30/opinion/christian-influencers-diet-culture-women.html (accessed September 19, 2025).
15 See Kristin Zeiler, "A Phenomenology of Excorporation, Bodily Alienation, and Resistance: Rethinking Sexed and Racialized Embodiment." *Hypatia* 28, no. 1 (2013), 69–84, https://doi.org/10.1111/j.1527-2001.2012.01305.x.
16 For more on the Miller tweet, see Kate Manne, *Unshrinking: How to Face Fatphobia* (Crown, 2014), 133.

Chapter 5. Body Positivity: A Revolution in Progress

1 Angela Davis, "Q&A Post Lecture at Southern Illinois University Carbondale," February 13, 2014, quoted by Jonathan Flowers in a post contemporaneously shared on Tumblr, https://www.tumblr.com/ninjaruski/76593432244/you-have-to-act-as-if-it-were-possible-to

(accessed September 21, 2025). For a history of this quotation and its misattributions, see Emilia Leese's "Revisiting an Angela Davis Quote," November 4, 2024, https://emisgoodeating.com/2024/11/04/revisiting-an-angela-davis-quote (accessed September 21, 2025).

2 Cheryl Frazier and Nadia Mehdi, "Forgetting Fatness: The Violent Co-optation of the Body Positivity Movement," *Debates in Aesthetics* 16, no. 1 (2021), 15.

3 Frazier and Mehdi, "Forgetting Fatness," 15.

4 Association for Size Diversity and Health, "About Health at Every Size."

5 Kate Manne, *Unshrinking: How to Face Fatphobia* (Crown, 2024), 202.

6 Mia Mingus, "Moving Toward the Ugly: A Politic Beyond Desirability," Femmes of Color Symposium Keynote Speech, Oakland, CA, August 21, 2011. For the text of her speech, see her blog, *Leaving Evidence*, https://leavingevidence.wordpress.com/2011/08/22/moving-toward-the-ugly-a-politic-beyond-desirability (accessed October 10, 2025).

7 This is an expression that Renee Engeln uses. See chapter 13 of *Beauty Sick: How the Cultural Obsession with Appearance Hurts Girls and Women* (HarperCollins, 2017).

8 Jessica Cwynar-Horta, "The Commodification of the Body Positive Movement on Instagram," *Stream* 8, no. 2 (2016): 36.

9 Sandra Bartky, "Narcissism, Femininity and Alienation," *Social Theory and Practice* 8, no. 2 (1982), 135.

10 Lizzo is quoted in Elyse Wanshel, "Lizzo: Body Positivity Has Been 'Co-Opted' and It's Not Helping Fat People." *HuffPost*, April 14, 2021, https://www.huffpost.com/entry/lizzo-body-positivity-has-been-co-opted-and-its-not-helping-fat-people_n_60773024e4b01654bb799710 (accessed September 20, 2025).

11 Frazier and Mehdi, "Forgetting Fatness," 14.

12 Anne Poirier is quoted in Charlotte Cowles's article, "Can 'Body Neutrality' Change the Way You Work Out? The Key to Staying Active Long Term May Be to Care Less about How You Look and More about How You Feel," *New York Times*, June 22, 2023, https://www.nytimes.com/2022/02/02/well/move/body-neutrality-exercise.html (accessed September 20, 2025).

13 I explore the criticism that body neutrality is ableist in my article "What Is Body Positivity? The Path from Shame to Pride," *Philosophical Topics*

47, no. 2 (Fall 2019): 113–27. See also Michelle Konstantinovsky's article "How Body Neutrality Can Help in Eating Disorder Recovery," Equip, September 11, 2025, https://equip.health/articles/body-image/body-neutrality-eating-disorder-recovery (accessed October 10, 2025).

14 Manne, *Unshrinking*, 204.

15 Manne, 205.

16 Manne, 205.

17 See Ann Saffi Biasetti, *Befriending Your Body: A Self-Compassionate Approach to Freeing Yourself from Disordered Eating* (Shambhala, 2018).

Chapter 6. Unbearable Weight: How the Pandemic Intensified Disordered Eating

1 Matthew Sanderson uses the example of a volcano in his presentation of the sublime in Kant. See his article, "Immanuel Kant's Theory of the Sublime," https://1000wordphilosophy.com/2023/11/11/kants-theory-of-the-sublime (accessed September 21, 2025).

2 I thank Elizabeth Scarbrough for her helpful explanation of the sublime, which she details in "What Makes Nature Beautiful?," *Introduction to Philosophy: Aesthetic Theory and Practice* (Rebus Community, 2021), https://press.rebus.community/intro-to-phil-aesthetics/chapter/what-makes-nature-beautiful (accessed September 21, 2025).

3 Sheila Lintott, "Sublime Hunger: A Consideration of Eating Disorders Beyond Beauty," *Hypatia* 18, no. 4 (2003), 80, http://www.jstor.org/stable/3810975.

4 Lintott, "Sublime Hunger," 79.

5 Marya Hornbacher, *Wasted: A Memoir of Anorexia and Bulimia* (HarperCollins, 1998), 125.

6 Hornbacher, *Wasted*, 125.

7 Lintott, "Sublime Hunger," 65.

8 Ruth Striegel Weissman and Philippa Hay, "People's Lived Experience with an Eating Disorder During the COVID-19 Pandemic: A Joint Virtual Issue of Research Published in Leading Eating Disorder Journals," *International Journal of Eating Disorders* 55, no. 2 (2022): 155–60, https://doi.org/10.1002/eat.23653.

9 National Institute of Health, "Risky Alcohol Use: An Epidemic Inside the COVID-19 Pandemic," 2003, https://covid19.nih.gov/news

-and-stories/risky-drinking-alcohol-use-epidemic-inside-covid-19 -pandemic. (This article is no longer available but was accessed October 20, 2023.)

10 Dora Bianchi et al., "Binge Eating as an Emotional Response to the COVID-19 Pandemic: A Sequential Mediation Model via the Impact of Events and Social Anxiety," *Journal of Eating Disord*ers 12 (2024): 209, https://doi.org/10.1186/s40337-024-01182-x.

11 See Emma Specter, *More, Please: On Food, Fat, Bingeing, Longing, and the Lust for "Enough"* (Harper, 2024).

12 David S. Freedman et al., "Weight Gain Among US Adults During the COVID-19 Pandemic Through May 2021," *Obesity* 30, no. 10 (2022), 2064–70, https://doi.org/10.1002/oby.23511.

13 American Psychological Association, "One Year On: Unhealthy Weight Gains, Increased Drinking Reported by Americans Coping with Pandemic Stress," March 11, 2021, https://www.apa.org/news/press/releases /2021/03/one-year-pandemic-stress; Elizabeth Pegg Frates, "Did We Really Gain Weight During the Pandemic?" Harvard School of Public Health, October 15, 2021, https://www.health.harvard.edu/blog/did -we-really-gain-weight-during-the-pandemic-202110052606.

14 Jade Portingale, Jesy Kenny, Matthew Fuller-Tyszkiewicz, and Isabel Krug, "Effects of Videoconferencing Use on Momentary Changes in Disordered Eating Urges, Body Dissatisfaction, and Mood," *European Eating Disorders Review* 32, no. 2 (2023): 201–14, https://doi.org /10.1002/erv.3036.

15 Rebecca Spigel et al., "Access to Care and Worsening Eating Disorder Symptomatology in Youth During the COVID-19 Pandemic," *Journal of Eating Disorders* 9, no. 1 (2021): 69, https://doi.org/10.1186/s40337 -021-00421-9.

16 Irina Jarvers et al. "Anorexia Nervosa During COVID-19: Loss of Personal Control and Alexithymia as Important Contributors to Symptomatology in Adolescent Girls," *Journal of Eating Disorders* 11 (2023): 180, https://doi.org/10.1186/s40337-023-00905-w.

17 Jarvers et al. "Anorexia Nervosa During COVID-19."

18 Jarvers et al. "Anorexia Nervosa During COVID-19."

19 "Alexithymia: Emotional Blindness," *Psychology Today*, n.d., https:// www.psychologytoday.com/us/basics/alexithymia (accessed September 21, 2025).

Chapter 7. Eating, Cooking, and the Ethics of Self-Care

1 Christopher Ziguras, *Self-Care: Embodiment, Personal Autonomy and the Shaping of Health Consciousness* (Routledge, 2004), 3.

2 Ziguras, *Self-Care*, 4.

3 Ziguras, *Self-Care*, 3.

4 Plato, *Apology*, trans. Benjamin Jowett (translation modified), https://classics.mit.edu/Plato/apology.html (accessed October 1, 2025).

5 See Emily Austin, *Living for Pleasure: An Epicurean Guide to Life* (Oxford University Press, 2023).

6 See Epicurus, *Letter to Menoeceus*, trans. Robert Drew Hicks, https://classics.mit.edu/Epicurus/menoec.html (accessed October 12, 2025).

7 Marcus Aurelius, *Meditations*, Book II, trans. George Long, https://classics.mit.edu/Antoninus/meditations.2.two.html (accessed October 1, 2025).

8 Jordan Kisner, "The Politics of Conspicuous Displays of Self-Care," *The New Yorker*, March 14, 2017, https://www.newyorker.com/culture/culture-desk/the-politics-of-selfcare.

9 Cartwright is quoted in Kisner's "The Politics of Conspicuous Displays of Self-Care."

10 Kisner, "Conspicuous Displays of Self-Care."

11 Kisner, "Conspicuous Displays of Self-Care."

12 Lorde, *A Burst of Light*, 130.

13 Kisner, "Conspicuous Displays of Self-Care."

14 Pooja Lakshmin, *Real Self-Care: A Transformative Program for Redefining Wellness* (Viking, 2023).

15 See chapter 7 of Ziguras's *Self-Care*.

16 See Ziguras, *Self-Care*, 124.

17 Ziguras quotes Lasch. See *Self-Care*, 124.

18 See W. E. B. Du Bois, *The Souls of Black Folk* https://www.gutenberg.org/files/408/408-h/408-h.htm (accessed August 1, 2025).

19 Myisha Cherry, "Solidarity Care: How to Take Care of Each Other in Times of Struggle," *Public Philosophy Journal* 3, no. 1 (2020), 3.

20 Cherry, "Solidarity Care," 10.

21 Audre Lorde, *Sister Outsider: Essays and Speeches by Audre Lorde* (Crossing, 2007), 112.

22 Mauren Salamon, "Feeding Body and Soul," Harvard Health Publishing, Harvard Medical School, https://www.health.harvard.edu/nutrition/feeding-body-and-soul (accessed October 12, 2025).
23 Salamon, "Feeding Body and Soul."
24 Evelyn Tribole, "Intuitive Eating in the Treatment of Eating Disorders: The Journey of Attunement," *Perspectives: A Professional Journal of The Renfrew Center Foundation* (Winter 2010), 12.
25 Tribole, "Intuitive Eating," 13.
26 See Casey Johnston, *A Physical Education: How I Escaped Diet Culture and Gained the Power of Lifting* (Grand Central, 2025).

Chapter 8. Resisting the Allure of Self-Objectification

1 Mia Beck Lichtenstein et al., "Compulsive Exercise: Links, Risks and Challenges Faced," *Psychology Research and Behavior Management* 10 (2017): 85–95, https://doi.org/10.2147/prbm.s113093.
2 Simone de Beauvoir, *The Prime of Life*, trans. Peter Green (Da Capo, 1994), 92.
3 Simone de Beauvoir, *The Second Sex*, trans. Constance Borde and Sheila Malovany-Chevallier (Vintage, 2011), 294.
4 Beauvoir, *Second Sex*, 295.
5 Beauvoir, *Second Sex*, 344.
6 Casey Johnston, *A Physical Education: How I Escaped Diet Culture and Gained the Power of Lifting* (Grand Central, 2025), 157.
7 Sonia Renee Taylor, *The Body Is Not an Apology: The Power of Radical Self-Love* (Berrett-Koehler, 2018), xi.
8 Taylor, *Body Is Not an Apology*, 11.
9 Taylor, 107.
10 Taylor, 108–9.
11 Taylor, 108.
12 Connie Sobczak, *Embody: Learning to Love Your Unique Body (And Quiet That Critical Voice!)* (Gürze Books, 2014), 109.
13 Sobczak, *Embody*, 109.
14 Sobczak, *Embody*, 109.
15 Elizabeth Barnes, *The Minority Body: A Theory of Disability* (Oxford University Press, 2016), 6.

16 Barnes, *Minority Body*, 6.
17 Barnes, *Minority Body*, 5.
18 Iris Marion Young, *On Female Body Experience: "Throwing Like a Girl" and Other Essays* (Oxford University Press, 2005), 36.
19 Young, *On Female Body Experience*, 40.
20 Young, *On Female Body Experience*, 45.
21 Sarah Grogan, *Body Image: Understanding Body Dissatisfaction in Men, Women and Children*, 4th ed. (Routledge), 224.
22 Grogan, *Body Image*, 224.
23 Grogan, *Body Image*, 224.
24 See the "Function over Form" chapter of *Beauty Sick: How the Cultural Obsession with Appearance Hurts Girls and Women* (HarperCollins, 2017).
25 Engeln, *Beauty Sick*, 298.
26 Engeln, *Beauty Sick*, 298.
27 Rachel H. Burgon, Jessica Beard, and Glenn Waller, "Body Image Concerns Across Different Sports and Sporting Levels: A Systematic Review and Meta-analysis," *Body Image* 46 (2023): 9–31, https://doi.org/10.1016/j.bodyim.2023.04.007.
28 Burgon, Beard, and Waller, "Body Image Concerns Across Different Sports."
29 Maher is quoted in Gina Vivinetto's article "Ilona Maher Gives 'Gentle but Firm' Reminder: 'It's OK to Exist in a Bigger Body,'" *Today*, February 27, 2025, https://www.today.com/health/mind-body/ilona-maher-body-image-reminder-rcna194059 (accessed September 21, 2025).
30 Burgon, Beard, and Waller, "Body Image Concerns Across Different Sports."
31 Taylor, *Body Is Not an Apology*, 100–102.
32 Jon Kabat-Zinn, *Coming to Our Senses: Healing Ourselves and the World Through Mindfulness* (Hyperion, 2005), 24.
33 Christopher K. Germer, *The Mindful Path to Self-Compassion: Freeing Yourself from Destructive Thoughts and Emotions* (Guilford, 2009), 37.
34 Germer, *Mindful Path to Self-Compassion*, 55, 43.
35 Germer, *Mindful Path to Self-Compassion*, 37.
36 William Edelglass, "The Bodhisattva Path: Santideva's Bodhicaryavatara," in *Buddhist Philosophy: Essential Readings*, ed. William Edelglass and Jay Garfield (Oxford University Press, 2009), 390.

37 Edelglass, "Bodhisattva Path," 390.
38 Jay Garfield, *Engaging Buddhism: Why It Matters to Philosophy* (Oxford University Press, 2015), 305.
39 Germer, *Mindful Path to Self-Compassion*, 49.

Chapter 9. Sensualism: Reigniting Pleasure and Desire In and For the Body

1 Karl Marx, "Estranged Labour," 1844, https://www.marxists.org/archive/marx/works/1844/manuscripts/labour.htm (accessed September 18, 2025).
2 Karl Marx, "Comments on James Mill, *Éléments D'économie Politique*," 1844, https://www.marxists.org/archive/marx/works/1844/james-mill (accessed September 18, 2025).
3 Leonard D. Katz, "Pleasure," *The Stanford Encyclopedia of Philosophy* (Winter 2016), ed. Edward N. Zalta, https://plato.stanford.edu/archives/win2016/entries/pleasure (accessed September 16, 2025).
4 Katz, "Pleasure."
5 Epictetus, *Enchiridion*, trans. Elizabeth Carter, https://classics.mit.edu/Epictetus/epicench.html (accessed September 17, 2025).
6 Marcus Aurelius, *Meditations*, Book VIII, trans. George Long, https://classics.mit.edu/Antoninus/meditations.8.eight.html (accessed September 17, 2025).
7 Marcus Aurelius, *Meditations*.
8 Epicurus, *Letter to Menoeceus*, trans. Robert Drew Hicks, https://classics.mit.edu/Epicurus/menoec.html (accessed September 14, 2025).
9 Epicurus, *Letter to Menoeceus*.
10 Epicurus.
11 Epicurus.
12 Lama Yeshe, *Introduction to Tantra: The Transformation of Desire*, ed. Jonatha Landaw (Wisdom, 2014), 17.
13 Lama Yeshe, *Introduction to Tantra*, 17.
14 These are Lama Yeshe's examples. See his *Introduction to Tantra*, 24.
15 Lama Yeshe, *Introduction to Tantra*, 25.
16 Lama Yeshe, *Introduction to Tantra*, 25.
17 See Thomas Moore, *A Religion of One's Own: A Guide to Creating a Personal Spirituality in a Secular World* (Penguin, 2015), 48.

18 Jenny Powers, "Outsourcing My Orgasm," *The Cut*, April 14, 2023, https://www.thecut.com/2023/04/outsourcing-my-orgasm.html (accessed September 22, 2025).

19 Powers, "Outsourcing My Orgasm."

20 Powers, "Outsourcing My Orgasm."

21 Meghan M. Gillen and Charlotte H. Markey, "A Review of Research Linking Body Image and Sexual Well-Being," *Body Image* 31 (2019): 294–301, https://doi.org/10.1016/j.bodyim.2018.12.004.

22 Zsolt Horvath et al., "Body Image, Orgasmic Response, and Sexual Relationship Satisfaction: Understanding Relationships and Establishing Typologies Based on Body Image Satisfaction," *Sexual Medicine* 8, no. 4 (December 2020): 740–51, https://doi.org/10.1016/j.esxm.2020.06.008.

23 Horvath et al., "Body Image, Orgasmic Response."

24 Emily Nagoski, *Come as You Are: The Surprising New Science That Will Transform Your Sex Life* (Simon & Schuster, 2021), 162.

25 Nagoski, *Come as You Are*, 162.

26 Nagoski, 161.

27 Nagoski, 162.

28 Nagoski, 163.

29 Nagoski, 180.

30 Nagoski, 180.

31 See chapter 9 of Engeln's *Beauty Sick*, "Media Literacy Is Not Enough," for a detailed discussion of the merits of media literacy.

32 For more about the history of this phrase, see BBC's reporting in "Kate Moss Regrets 'Nothing Tastes As Good As Skinny Feels' Comment," September 14, 2018, https://www.bbc.com/news/newsbeat-45522714 (accessed October 15, 2025).

33 Jade Biggs, "Former Supermodel Kate Moss Reflects on Her Infamous Line: 'Nothing Tastes As Good As Skinny Feels,'" *Cosmopolitan UK*, July 25, 2022, https://www.cosmopolitan.com/uk/body/health/a40703565/kate-moss-reflects-nothing-tastes-as-good-as-skinny-feels (accessed October 15, 2025).

34 Plato, *Philebus*, trans. Benjamin Jowett, https://www.gutenberg.org/files/1744/1744-h/1744-h.htm (accessed October 12, 2025).

35 Plato, *Philebus.*

36 Patricia Marechal, "Plato on False Pleasures and False Passions," *Apeiron* 55, no. 2 (2022), 302, https://doi.org/10.1515/apeiron-2020-0090.

37 See chapter 4 of Manne's *Unshrinking*, "Demoralizing Fatness," for more information about the "moral panic" around obesity.

38 Breanne Fahs and Denise Delgado, "The Specter of Excess: Race, Class, and Gender in Women's Body Hair Narratives," in *Embodied Resistance: Challenging the Norms, Breaking the Rules*, ed. Chris Bobel and Samantha Kwan (Vanderbilt University Press, 2011), 23.

39 Nathaniel C. Pyle and Noa Logan Klein, "Fat. Hairy. Sexy: Contesting Stands of Beauty and Sexuality in the Gay Community," in *Embodied Resistance: Challenging the Norms, Breaking the Rules*, 82.

40 Pyle and Klein, "Fat. Hairy. Sexy," 84.

41 Pyle and Klein, 83.

42 Pyle and Klein, 85.

43 Pyle and Klein, 86.

44 For an account of these workshops, see Betty Dodson's *Sex for One: The Joy of Selfloving* (Harmony Books, 1996).

45 Céline Leboeuf, "Anatomy of the Thigh Gap," *Feminist Philosophy Quarterly* 5, no. 1, 20.

Chapter 10. Remaking the World

1 Simone de Beauvoir, *The Second Sex*, trans. Constance Borde and Sheila Malovany-Chevallier (Vintage, 2011), 46 (translation modified).

2 Martin Heidegger, *Being and Time*, trans. John Macquarrie and Edward Robinson (Harper & Row, 1962), 93.

3 Martin Heidegger, *History of the Concept of Time*, trans. Theodore Kisiel (Indiana University Press, 2009), 166.

4 Heidegger, *History of the Concept of Time*, 166.

5 See Heidegger, *Being and Time*, Section 17.

6 See Heidegger, *Being and Time*, Section 15.

7 Heidegger, *Being and Time*, 116.

8 See Heidegger, *Being and Time*, Section 18.

9 María Lugones, "Playfulness, 'World'-Travelling, and Loving Perception," *Hypatia* 2, no. 2 (1987): 3–19, http://www.jstor.org/stable/3810013, 3.

10 Lugones, "Playfulness, 'World'-Travelling, and Loving Perception," 10.
11 Lugones, 11.
12 Lugones, 17.
13 Lugones, 17.
14 Lugones, 17.
15 Lugones, 3.
16 Alia Al-Saji, "A Phenomenology of Hesitation: Interrupting Racializing Habits of Seeing," in *Living Alterities: Phenomenology, Embodiment, and Race*, ed. Emily S. Lee (SUNY Press, 2014), 149.
17 Lugones, "Playfulness, 'World'-Travelling, and Loving Perception," 18.
18 Leo Tolstoy, *A Confession*, trans. Aylmer Maude (Dover, 2005), 17.
19 A. W. Eaton, "Taste in Bodies and Fat Oppression," in *Body Aesthetics*, ed. Sherri Irvin (Oxford University Press, 2016).
20 These are Aristotle's words quoted in Eaton, "Taste in Bodies and Fat Oppression," 49.
21 Eaton, "Taste in Bodies and Fat Oppression," 54.
22 Eaton, "Taste in Bodies and Fat Oppression," 56.
23 Renee Engeln, *Beauty Sick: How the Cultural Obsession with Appearance Hurts Girls and Women* (HarperCollins, 2017), 202.
24 Jean-Paul Sartre, *Existentialism Is a Humanism*, trans. Carol Macomber (Yale University Press, 2007), 24–25.
25 Friedrich Nietzsche, *The Anti-Christ, Ecce Homo, Twilight of the Idols and Other Writings*, ed. Aaron Ridley and Judith Norman (Cambridge University Press, 2005), 87.
26 Dacher Keltner, *Awe: The New Science of Everyday Wonder and How It Can Transform Your Life* (Penguin, 2023), 7.
27 Keltner, *Awe*, 127–28.
28 Keltner, 128.
29 Keltner, 134–35.
30 Helen De Cruz, *Wonderstruck: How Wonder and Awe Shape the Way We Think* (Princeton University Press, 2024), 4.
31 De Cruz, *Wonderstruck*, 4.
32 De Cruz, *Wonderstruck*, 5.
33 Viren Swami, David Barron, and Adrian Furnham, "Exposure to Natural Environments, and Photographs of Natural Environments, Promotes More Positive Body Image," *Body Image* 24 (2018): 82–94, https://doi.org/10.1016/j.bodyim.2017.12.006.

34 Viren Swami, "Associations Between Nature Exposure and Body Image: A Critical, Narrative Review of the Evidence," *Acta Psychologica* 248 (2024), https://doi.org/10.1016/j.actpsy.2024.104355.

35 Swami, "Associations Between Nature Exposure and Body Image."

36 Lisa Blake, "Why This Colorado Photographer Thinks More People Should Be Nude in Nature," 5280, September 12, 2024, https://5280.com/why-this-colorado-photographer-thinks-more-people-should-be-nude-in-nature (accessed September 28, 2025).

Epilogue

1 Simone de Beauvoir, *The Second Sex,* trans. Constance Borde and Sheila Malovany-Chevallier (Vintage, 2011), 3.

2 Audre Lorde, "The Uses of Anger," *Women Studies Quarterly* (CUNY Academic Works), 10.

Bibliography

Ahmad, Meher, and Jessica Grose. "Why the Right Is Obsessed With Thinness: When Diet Culture Meets Conservative Morality." *New York Times*, July 30, 2025. https://www.nytimes.com/2025/07/30/opinion/christian-influencers-diet-culture-women.html (accessed September 19, 2025).

Al-Saji, Alia. "A Phenomenology of Hesitation: Interrupting Racializing Habits of Seeing." In *Living Alterities: Phenomenology, Embodiment, and Race*, edited by Emily S. Lee. SUNY Press, 2014.

American Psychological Association. "One Year On: Unhealthy Weight Gains, Increased Drinking Reported by Americans Coping with Pandemic Stress." March 11, 2021. https://www.apa.org/news/press/releases/2021/03/one-year-pandemic-stress (accessed September 21, 2025).

Aristotle. *Nicomachean Ethics*. Translated by W. D. Ross. Internet Classics Archive. https://classics.mit.edu/Aristotle/nicomachaen.html.

Association for Size Diversity and Health. "About Health at Every Size." https://asdah.org/haes (accessed September 20, 2025).

Aurelius, Marcus. *Meditations*. Translated by George Long. Internet Classics Archive. https://classics.mit.edu/Antoninus/meditations.html (accessed October 1, 2025).

Austin, Emily. *Living for Pleasure: An Epicurean Guide to Life*. Oxford University Press, 2023.

Baker Hyde, Phoebe. *The Beauty Experiment*. Da Capo, 2013.

Barakat, Sarah, Siân A. McLean, Emma Bryant, Anvi Le, Peta Marks, National Eating Disorder Research Consortium, Stephen Touyz, and Sarah Maguire. "Risk Factors for Eating Disorders: Findings from a Rapid Review." *Journal of Eating Disorders* 11, no. 8 (2023). https://jeatdisord.biomedcentral.com/articles/10.1186/s40337-022-00717-4 (accessed September 13, 2025).

Barnes, Elizabeth. *The Minority Body: A Theory of Disability*. Oxford University Press, 2016.

Bartky, Sandra. "Narcissism, Femininity and Alienation." *Social Theory and Practice* 8, no. 2 (Summer 1982): 127–43.

Basberg Neumann, Cecilie. "A Dangerous Subject: The Fashion Model and the Beauty/Narcissism Double Bind," *Hypatia* 32, no. 2 (2017): 380–96.

Batista, Maya, Lana Žigić Antić, Orjena Žaja, Trpimir Jakovina, and Ivan Begovac. "Predictors of Eating Disorder Risk in Anorexia Nervosa Adolescents." *Acta Clinica Croatica* 57, no. 3 (2018): 399–410. https://doi.org/10.20471/acc.2018.57.03.01.

Bauer, Nancy. "Lady Power." *New York Times*, June 20, 2010. https://archive.nytimes.com/opinionator.blogs.nytimes.com/2010/06/20/lady-power (accessed August 15, 2025).

Bauer, Nancy. "Simone de Beauvoir on the Allure of Self-Objectification." In *Feminist Metaphysics: Explorations in the Ontology of Sex, Gender and the Self*, edited by Charlotte Witt. Springer, 2011.

BBC. "Kate Moss Regrets 'Nothing Tastes As Good As Skinny Feels' Comment." BBC, September 14, 2018. https://www.bbc.com/news/newsbeat-45522714 (accessed October 15, 2025).

Beauvoir, Simone de. *The Prime of Life.* Translated by Peter Green. Da Capo, 1994.

Beauvoir, Simone de. *The Second Sex.* Translated by Constance Borde and Sheila Malovany-Chevallier. Vintage Books, 2011.

Beck Lichtenstein, Mia, Cecilie Juul Hinze, Bolette Emborg, Freja Thomsen, and Simone Daugaard Hemmingsen. "Compulsive Exercise: Links, Risks and Challenges Faced." *Psychology Research and Behavior Management* 10 (2017): 85–95. https://doi.org/10.2147/prbm.s113093.

Bianchi, Dora, Daniela Di Tata, Anna Di Norcia, Sara Pompii, Laura Maria Fatta, and Fiorenzo Laghi. "Binge Eating as an Emotional Response to the COVID-19 Pandemic: A Sequential Mediation Model via the Impact of Events and Social Anxiety." *Journal of Eating Disorders* 12, article 209 (2024). https://doi.org/10.1186/s40337-024-01182-x.

Diggs, Jade. "Former Supermodel Kate Moss Reflects on Her Infamous Line: 'Nothing Tastes As Good As Skinny Feels.'" *Cosmopolitan UK*, July 25, 2022. https://www.cosmopolitan.com/uk/body/health/a40703565/kate-moss-reflects-nothing-tastes-as-good-as-skinny-feels (accessed October 15, 2025).

Blake, Lisa. "Why This Colorado Photographer Thinks More People Should Be Nude in Nature." 5280, September 12, 2024. https://5280.com/why-this-colorado-photographer-thinks-more-people-should-be-nude-in-nature (accessed September 28, 2025).

Bordo, Susan. *Unbearable Weight: Feminism, Western Culture, and the Body.* University of California Press, 1993.

Bourdieu, Pierre. *Distinction: A Social Critique of the Judgement of Taste.* Translated by Richard Nice. Harvard University Press, 1984.

Bourdieu, Pierre, and Loïc Wacquant. *An Invitation to Reflexive Sociology.* University of Chicago Press, 1992.

Breton, Édith, Rachel Dufour, Sylvana M. Côté, Lise Dubois, Frank Vitaro, Michel Boivin, Richard E. Tremblay, and Linda Booij. "Developmental Trajectories of Eating Disorder Symptoms: A Longitudinal Study from Early Adolescence to Young Adulthood." *Journal of Eating Disorders* 10, no. 1 (2022). https://doi.org/10.1186/s40337-022-00603-z.

Burgon, Rachel, Jessica Beard, and Glenn Waller. "Body Image Concerns Across Different Sports and Sporting Levels: A Systematic Review and Meta-analysis." *Body Image* 46 (September 2023): 9–31. https://doi.org/10.1016/j.bodyim.2023.04.007.

Butler, Judith. *Gender Trouble: Feminism and the Subversion of Identity.* Routledge, 1990.

Cahill, Ann J. "Feminist Pleasure and Feminine Beautification." *Hypatia* 18, no. 4 (2003), 42–64.

Chernin, Kim. *The Obsession: Reflections on the Tyranny of Slenderness.* Harper & Row, 1981.

Cherry, Myisha. "Solidarity Care: How to Take Care of Each Other in Times of Struggle." *Public Philosophy Journal* 3, no. 1 (2020): 1–12. https://doi.org/10.25335/PPJ.3.1-4.

Cowles, Charlotte. "Can 'Body Neutrality' Change the Way You Work Out? The Key to Staying Active Long-Term May Be to Care Less About How You Look and More About How You Feel." *New York Times*, June 22, 2023. https://www.nytimes.com/2022/02/02/well/move/body-neutrality-exercise.html (accessed September 20, 2025).

Cwynar-Horta, Jessica. "The Commodification of the Body Positive Movement on Instagram." *Stream* 8, no. 2 (2016): 36–56.

Davis, Angela. "Q&A Post Lecture at Southern Illinois University Carbondale." Quoted by Jonathan Flowers in a Tumblr post. February 13, 2014. https://www.tumblr.com/ninjaruski/76593432244/you-have-to-act-as-if-it-were-possible-to (accessed September 21, 2025).

De Cruz, Helen. *Wonderstruck: How Wonder and Awe Shape the Way We Think.* Princeton University Press, 2024.

Dodson, Betty. *Sex for One: The Joy of Selfloving.* Harmony Books, 1996.

Dolezal, Luna. *The Body and Shame: Phenomenology, Feminism, and the Socially Shaped Body*. Lexington Books, 2015.

Du Bois, W. E. B. *The Souls of Black Folk.* Project Gutenberg, 2021: https://www.gutenberg.org/files/408/408-h/408-h.htm (accessed August 1, 2025).

Eaton, A. W. "Taste in Bodies and Fat Oppression." In *Body Aesthetics*, edited by Sherri Irvin. Oxford University Press, 2016.

Edelglass, William. "The Bodhisattva Path: Santideva's Bodhicaryavatara." In *Buddhist Philosophy: Essential Readings*, edited by William Edelglass and Jay Garfield. Oxford University Press, 2009.

Engeln, Renee. *Beauty Sick: How the Cultural Obsession with Appearance Hurts Girls and Women*. HarperCollins, 2017.

Epictetus. *Enchiridion.* Translated by Elizabeth Carter. Internet Classics Archive. https://classics.mit.edu/Epictetus/epicench.html (accessed September 17, 2025).

Epicurus. *Letter to Menoeceus.* Translated by Robert Drew Hicks. Internet Classics Archive. https://classics.mit.edu/Epicurus/menoec.html (accessed October 1, 2025).

Etcoff, Nancy. *Survival of the Prettiest: The Science of Beauty*. Anchor Books, 1999.

Fahs, Breanne, and Denise Delgado. "The Specter of Excess: Race, Class, and Gender in Women's Body Hair Narratives." In *Embodied Resistance: Challenging the Norms, Breaking the Rules*, edited by Chris Bobel and Samantha Kwan. Vanderbilt University Press, 2011.

Forney, K. Jean, Teresa Schwendler, and Rose Marie Ward. "Examining Similarities in Eating Pathology, Negative Affect, and Perfectionism Among Peers: A Social Network Analysis." *Appetite* (2019): 236–43. https://doi.org/10.1016/j.appet.2019.03.013.

Frazier, Cheryl. "Beauty Labor as a Tool to Resist Antifatness," *Hypatia* 38, no. 2 (2023), 231–50. https://doi.org/10.1017/hyp.2023.22.

Frazier, Cheryl, and Nadia Mehdi. "Forgetting Fatness: The Violent Co-optation of the Body Positivity Movement." *Debates in Aesthetics* 16, no. 1 (2021): 13–28.

Freedman, David S., Lyudmyla Kompaniyets, Carrie Daymont, Lixia Zhao, and Heidi M. Blanck. "Weight Gain Among US Adults During the COVID-19 Pandemic Through May 2021." *Obesity* 30, no. 10 (2022): 2064–70. https://doi.org/10.1002/oby.23511.

Frye, Marilyn. *The Politics of Reality: Essays in Feminist Theory*. Crossing, 1983.

Future Market Insights. "Hair Straightener Market," updated September 8, 2025. https://www.futuremarketinsights.com/reports/hair-straightener-market (accessed October 8, 2025).

Garfield, Jay. *Engaging Buddhism: Why It Matters to Philosophy.* Oxford University Press, 2015.

Gay, Roxane. *Hunger: A Memoir of (My) Body.* HarperCollins, 2017.

Germer, Christopher K. *The Mindful Path to Self-Compassion: Freeing Yourself from Destructive Thoughts and Emotions.* Guilford, 2009.

Gillen, Meghan M., and Charlotte H. Markey. "A Review of Research Linking Body Image and Sexual Well-Being." *Body Image* 31 (2019): 294–301. https://doi.org/10.1016/j.bodyim.2018.12.004.

Global Market Insights. "Hair Straightener Market Size," December 2025. https://www.gminsights.com/industry-analysis/hair-straightener-market (accessed October 7, 2025).

Gorrell, Sasha, and Stuart B. Murray, "Eating Disorders in Males." *Child and Adolescent Psychiatric Clinics of North America* 28, no. 4 (2019): 641–51.

Grogan, Sarah. *Body Image: Understanding Body Dissatisfaction in Men, Women and Children*, 4th ed. Routledge, 2022.

Heidegger, Martin. *Being and Time.* Translated by John Macquarrie and Edward Robinson. Harper & Row, 1962.

Heidegger, Martin. *History of the Concept of Time.* Translated by Theodore Kisiel. Indiana University Press, 2009.

Hickman, Timothy. "Heroin Chic: The Visual Culture of Narcotic Addiction." *Third Text* 16, no. 2 (2002): 119–36. https://doi.org/10.1080/09528820210138272.

Hornbacher, Marya. *Wasted: A Memoir of Anorexia and Bulimia.* HarperCollins, 1998.

Horvath, Zsolt, Betina Hodt Smith, Dorottya Sal, Krisztina Hevesi, and David L. Rowland. "Body Image, Orgasmic Response, and Sexual Relationship Satisfaction: Understanding Relationships and Establishing Typologies Based on Body Image Satisfaction." *Sexual Medicine* 8, no. 4 (December 2020): 740–51. https://doi.org/10.1016/j.esxm.2020.06.008.

Ireland, Corydon. "Fijian Girls Succumb to Western Dysmorphia." *Harvard Gazette*, March 19, 2009. https://news.harvard.edu/gazette/story/2009/03/fijian-girls-succumb-to-western-dysmorphia (accessed September 13, 2025).

Jarvers, Irina, Angelika Ecker, Daniel Schleicher, Stephanie Kandsperger, Alexandra Otto, and Romuald Brunner. "Anorexia Nervosa During COVID-19: Loss of Personal Control and Alexithymia as Important Contributors to Symptomatology in Adolescent Girls." *Journal of Eating Disorders* 11, article 180 (2023). https://doi.org/10.1186/s40337-023-00905-w.

Johnston, Casey. *A Physical Education: How I Escaped Diet Culture and Gained the Power of Lifting.* Grand Central, 2025.

Kabat-Zinn, Jon. *Coming to Our Senses: Healing Ourselves and the World Through Mindfulness.* Hyperion, 2005.

Katz, Leonard D. "Pleasure." *The Stanford Encyclopedia of Philosophy* (Winter 2016), edited by Edward N. Zalta. https://plato.stanford.edu/archives/win2016/entries/pleasure (accessed September 16, 2025).

Keltner, Dacher. *Awe: The New Science of Everyday Wonder and How It Can Transform Your Life.* Penguin, 2023.

Kendal, Sarah, Sue Kirk, Rebecca Elvey, Roger Catchpole, and Steven Pryjmachuk. "How a Moderated Online Discussion Forum Facilitates Support for Young People with Eating Disorders." *Health Expectations* 20 (2016): 98–111. https://doi.org/10.1111/hex.12439.

Kisner, Jordan. "The Politics of Conspicuous Displays of Self-Care." *New Yorker*, March 14, 2017. https://www.newyorker.com/culture/culture-desk/the-politics-of-selfcare.

Konstantinovsky, Michelle. "How Body Neutrality Can Help in Eating Disorder Recovery." Equip, September 11, 2025. https://equip.health/articles/body-image/body-neutrality-eating-disorder-recovery (accessed October 10, 2025).

Kontele, Ioanna, Stella Saripanagiotou, Agni Maria Papadopoulou, Evangelos Zoumbaneas, and Tonia Vassilakou. "Parental Dieting and Correlation with Disordered Eating Behaviours in Adolescents: A Narrative Review." *Adolescents* 3, no. 3 (2023): 538–49. https://doi.org/10.3390/adolescents3030038.

Lakshmin, Pooja. *Real Self-Care: A Transformative Program for Redefining Wellness.* Viking, 2023.

Lama Yeshe. *Introduction to Tantra: The Transformation of Desire.* Edited by Jonatha Landaw. Wisdom Publications, 2014.

Langton, Rae. *Sexual Solipsism: Philosophical Essays on Pornography and Objectification.* Oxford University Press, 2001.

Leboeuf, Céline. "Anatomy of the Thigh Gap." *Feminist Philosophy Quarterly* 5, no. 1 (2019): 1–22. https://doi.org/10.5206/fpq/2019.1.7312.

Leboeuf, Céline. "What Is Body Positivity? The Path from Shame to Pride." *Philosophical Topics* 47, no. 2 (Fall 2019): 113–27. https://doi.org/10.5206/fpq/2019.1.7312.

Leese, Emilia. "Revisiting an Angela Davis Quote," November 4, 2024. https://emisgoodeating.com/2024/11/04/revisiting-an-angela-davis-quote (accessed September 21, 2025).

Lintott, Sheila. "Sublime Hunger: A Consideration of Eating Disorders Beyond Beauty." *Hypatia* 18, no. 4 (2003): 65–86. http://www.jstor.org/stable/3810975.

Lorde, Audre. *A Burst of Light and Other Essays.* Ixia, 2017.

Lorde, Audre. *Sister Outsider: Essays and Speeches by Audre Lorde.* Crossing, 2007.

Lorde, Audre. "The Uses of Anger." *Women Studies Quarterly* (CUNY Academic Works): 6–10.

Lugones, María. "Playfulness, 'World'-Travelling, and Loving Perception." *Hypatia* 2, no. 2 (1987): 3–19. http://www.jstor.org/stable/3810013.

Manne, Kate. *Unshrinking: How to Face Fatphobia*. Crown, 2024.

Marechal, Patricia. "Plato on False Pleasures and False Passions." *Apeiron* 55, no. 2 (2022): 281–304. https://doi.org/10.1515/apeiron-2020-0090.

Marx, Karl. "Comments on James Mill, *Éléments D'économie Politique.*" 1844. https://www.marxists.org/archive/marx/works/1844/james-mill (accessed September 18, 2025).

Marx, Karl. "Estranged Labour." 1844. https://www.marxists.org/archive/marx/works/1844/manuscripts/labour.htm (accessed September 18, 2025).

Micali, Nadia, Maria G. Martini, Jennifer J. Thomas, Kamryn T. Eddy, Radha Kothari, Ellie Russell, Cynthia M. Bulik, and Janet Treasure. "Lifetime and 12-Month Prevalence of Eating Disorders Amongst Women in Mid-Life: A Population-Based Study of Diagnoses and Risk Factors." *BMC Medicine* 15, no. 12 (2017). https://doi.org/10.1186/s12916-016-0766-4.

Mingus, Mia. "Moving Toward the Ugly: A Politic Beyond Desirability." Femmes of Color Symposium Keynote Speech, Oakland, CA, August 21, 2011. Leaving Evidence, August 22, 2011. https://leavingevidence.wordpress.com/2011/08/22/moving-toward-the-ugly-a-politic-beyond-desirability (accessed October 10, 2025).

Moore, Thomas. *A Religion of One's Own: A Guide to Creating a Personal Spirituality in a Secular World.* Penguin, 2015.

Nagoski, Emily. *Come as You Are: The Surprising New Science That Will Transform Your Sex Life.* Simon & Schuster, 2021.

National Association of Anorexia Nervosa and Associated Disorders. "Eating Disorder Statistics," n.d. https://anad.org/eating-disorder-statistic (accessed August 1, 2025).

National Institutes of Health. "Risky Alcohol Use: An Epidemic Inside the COVID-19 Pandemic." 2023. https://covid19.nih.gov/news-and-stories/risky-drinking-alcohol-use-epidemic-inside-covid-19-pandemic (accessed October 20, 2023; no longer available).

Neumark-Sztainer, Dianne, Melanie M. Wall, Chen Chen, Nicole I. Larson, Mary J. Christoph, and Nancy E. Sherwood. "Eating, Activity, and Weight-Related Problems from Adolescence to Adulthood." *American Journal of Preventive Medicine* 55, no. 2 (2018): 133–41 https://doi.org/10.1016/j.amepre.2018.04.032.

Nietzsche, Friedrich. *The Anti-Christ, Ecce Homo, Twilight of the Idols and Other Writings*, edited by Aaron Ridley and Judith Norman. Cambridge University Press, 2005.

Norsigian, Judy, Vilunya Diskin, Paula Doress-Worters, Jane Pincus, Wendy Sanford, and Norma Swenson. "The Boston Women's Health Book Collective and 'Our Bodies, Ourselves': A Brief History and Reflection." https://ourbodiesourselves.org/impact-influence/the-boston-womens-health-book-collective-and-our-bodies-ourselves-a-brief-history-and-reflection (accessed October 4, 2025).

Pegg Frates, Elizabeth. "Did We Really Gain Weight During the Pandemic?" Harvard School of Public Health, October 15, 2021. https://www.health.harvard.edu/blog/did-we-really-gain-weight-during-the-pandemic-202110052606 (accessed August 27, 2025).

Pisetsky, Emily M., Laura M. Thornton, Paul Lichtenstein, Nancy L. Pedersen, and Cynthia M. Bulik. "Suicide Attempts in Women with Eating Disorders." *Journal of Abnormal Psychology* 122, no. 4 (2013): 1042–56. https://doi.org/10.1037/a0034902.

Plato. *Apology.* Translated by Benjamin Jowett. https://classics.mit.edu/Plato/apology.html (accessed October 1, 2025).

Plato. *Philebus.* Translated by Benjamin Jowett. Project Gutenberg, 2013. https://www.gutenberg.org/files/1744/1744-h/1744-h.htm (accessed October 12, 2025).

Portingale, Jade, Jesy Kenny, Matthew Fuller-Tyszkiewicz, and Isabel Krug. "Effects of Videoconferencing Use on Momentary Changes in Disordered Eating Urges, Body Dissatisfaction, and Mood." *European Eating Disorders Review* 32, no. 2 (2023): 201–14. https://doi.org/10.1002/erv.3036.

Powers, Jenny. "Outsourcing My Orgasm." The Cut, April 14, 2023. https://www.thecut.com/2023/04/outsourcing-my-orgasm.html (accessed September 22, 2025

Psychology Today. "Alexithymia: Emotional Blindness." https://www.psychologytoday.com/us/basics/alexithymia (accessed September 21, 2025).

Pursey, Kirrilly M., Tracy L. Burrows, Daniel Barker, Melissa Hart, and Susan J. Paxton. "Disordered Eating, Body Image Concerns, and Weight Control Behaviors in Primary School Aged Children: A Systematic Review and Meta-analysis of Universal–Selective Prevention Interventions." *International Journal of Eating Disorders* 54, no. 10 (2021): 1730–65. https://doi.org/10.1002/eat.23571 (accessed September 13, 2025).

Pyle, Nathaniel C. and Noa Logan Klein. "Fat. Hairy. Sexy: Contesting Stands of Beauty and Sexuality in the Gay Community." In *Embodied Resistance: Challenging the Norms, Breaking the Rules*, edited by Chris Bobel and Samantha Kwan. Vanderbilt University Press, 2011.

Rizzo, Mary. "Embodying Withdrawal: Abjection and the Popularity of Heroin Chic." *Michigan Feminist Studies* 15 (2001). http://hdl.handle.net/2027/spo.ark5583.0015.004 (accessed September 15, 2025).

Saffi Biasetti, Ann. *Befriending Your Body: A Self-Compassionate Approach to Freeing Yourself from Disordered Eating.* Shambhala, 2018.

Salamon, Maureen. "Feeding Body and Soul." Harvard Health Publishing, Harvard Medical School, August 1, 2023. https://www.health.harvard.edu/nutrition/feeding-body-and-soul (accessed October 12, 2025).

Sanderson, Matthew. "Immanuel Kant's Theory of the Sublime." 1000-Word Philosophy: An Introductory Anthology, November 11, 2023. https://1000wordphilosophy.com/2023/11/11/kants-theory-of-the-sublime (accessed September 21, 2025).

Sartre, Jean-Paul. *Existentialism Is a Humanism.* Translated by Carol Macomber. Yale University Press, 2007.

Scarbrough, Elizabeth. "What Makes Nature Beautiful?" In *Introduction to Philosophy: Aesthetic Theory and Practice.* Rebus Community, 2021. https://press.rebus.community/intro-to-phil-aesthetics/chapter/what-makes-nature-beautiful.

Scheldrup, Gavin. "The Ozempic Era." Medical University of South Carolina, August 29, 2024. https://gradstudies.musc.edu/about/blog/2024/08/the-ozempic-era (accessed August 25, 2025).

Shakin, Chloe W. "Chin Hair, Laundry, Your Opinion: Women in Menopause Don't Care." *New York Times.* June 24, 2025. https://www.nytimes.com/2025/06/24/well/menopause-melani-sanders-club.html (accessed July 25, 2025).

Siegel, Jaclyn A., Virginia Ramseyer Winter, and Mackenzie Cook. "'It Really Presents a Struggle for Females, Especially My Little Girl': Exploring Fathers' Experiences Discussing Body Image with Their Young Daughters." *Body Image* 36 (2021): 84–94. https://doi.org/10.1016/j.bodyim.2020.11.001 (accessed January 15, 2023).

Sobczak, Connie. *Embody: Learning to Love Your Unique Body (And Quiet That Critical Voice!).* Gürze Books, 2014.

Specter, Emma. *More, Please: On Food, Fat, Bingeing, Longing, and the Lust for "Enough."* Harper, 2024.

Spencer-Oatey, Heather. *Culturally Speaking. Culture, Communication and Politeness Theory,* 2nd ed. Continuum, 2008.

Spigel, Rebecca, Jessica A. Lin, Carly E. Milliren, Melissa Freizinger, Julia A. Vitagliano, Elizabeth R. Woods, Sara F. Forman, and Tracy K. Richmond. "Access to Care and Worsening Eating Disorder Symptomatology in Youth During the COVID-19 Pandemic." *Journal of Eating Disorders* 9, no. 1 (2021): 69. https://doi.org/10.1186/s40337-021-00421-9.

Statista. "Most Popular Social Networks Worldwide as of February 2025, by Number of Monthly Active Users." https://www.statista.com/statistics/272014/global-social-networks-ranked-by-number-of-users (accessed August 26, 2025)

Striegel Weissman, Ruth, and Philippa Hay. "People's Lived Experience with an Eating Disorder During the COVID-19 Pandemic: A Joint Virtual Issue of Research Published in Leading Eating Disorder Journals."

International Journal of Eating Disorders 55, no. 2 (2022): 155–60. https://doi.org/10.1002/eat.23653.
Strings, Sabrina. *Fearing the Black Body: The Racial Origins of Fat Phobia.* New York University Press, 2019.
Swami, Viren, David Barron, and Adrian Furnham. "Exposure to Natural Environments, and Photographs of Natural Environments, Promotes More Positive Body Image." *Body Image* 24 (2018): 82–94. https://doi.org/10.1016/j.bodyim.2017.12.006.
Taylor, Sonia Renee. *The Body Is Not an Apology: The Power of Radical Self-Love.* Berrett-Koehler, 2018.
Thomas, Jennifer, and Jenni Schaefer, *Almost Anorexic: Is My (or My Loved One's) Relationship with Food a Problem?* Hazelden, 2013.
Tolstoy, Leo. *A Confession.* Translated by Aylmer Maude. Dover, 2005.
Tribole, Evelyn. "Intuitive Eating in the Treatment of Eating Disorders: The Journey of Attunement." *Perspectives: A Professional Journal of The Renfrew Center Foundation* (Winter 2010): 11–14.
van Eeden, Annelies, Daphne van Hoeken, and Hans Hoek. "Incidence, Prevalence and Mortality of Anorexia Nervosa and Bulimia Nervosa." *Current Opinion in Psychiatry* 34, no. 6 (2021): 515–24. https://doi.org/10.1097/YCO.0000000000000739.
Vivinetto, Gina. "Ilona Maher Gives 'Gentle but Firm' Reminder: 'It's OK to Exist in a Bigger Body.'" *Today*, February 27, 2025. https://www.today.com/health/mind-body/ilona-maher-body-image-reminder-rcna194059 (accessed September 21, 2025).
Wanshel, Emily. "Lizzo: Body Positivity Has Been 'Co-Opted' and It's Not Helping Fat People." *HuffPost*, April 14, 2021. https://www.huffpost.com/entry/lizzo-body-positivity-has-been-co-opted-and-its-not-helping-fat-people_n_60773024e4b01654bb799710 (accessed September 20, 2025).
Whyte, Hilary E. A., S. M. Findlay, and Canadian Paediatric Society, Adolescent Health Committee. "Dieting in Adolescence." *Paediatrics & Child Health* 9, no. 7 (September 2004): 487–91. https://doi.org/10.1093/pch/9.7.487 (accessed September 12, 2025).
Widdows, Heather. *Perfect Me: Beauty as an Ethical Ideal.* Princeton University Press, 2018.
Wissinger, Elizabeth. *This Year's Model: Fashion, Media, and the Making of Glamour.* New York University Press, 2015.

Wolf, Naomi. *The Beauty Myth: How Images of Beauty Are Used Against Women*. HarperPerennial, 2002.

World Health Organization. "Moderate and Severe Thinness, Underweight, Overweight, Obesity." https://apps.who.int/nutrition/landscape/help.aspx?menu=0&helpid=420 (accessed September 11, 2025).

Young, Iris Marion. *On Female Body Experience: "Throwing Like a Girl" and Other Essays*. Oxford University Press, 2005.

Zeiler, Kristin. "A Phenomenology of Excorporation, Bodily Alienation, and Resistance: Rethinking Sexed and Racialized Embodiment." *Hypatia* 28, no. 1 (2013): 69–84. https://doi.org/10.1111/j.1527-2001.2012.01305.x.

Ziguras, Christopher. *Self-Care: Embodiment, Personal Autonomy and the Shaping of Health Consciousness*. Routledge, 2004.

Acknowledgments

Just as combating the tyranny of thinness is never done alone, so too I could never have written this book without the support of others.

Words can hardly convey the debt I owe to Nancy Bauer, who taught me the value of feminist philosophy and instilled in me a passion for Simone de Beauvoir. I thank you for these lessons and for shoring me up during the final stages of my doctoral dissertation. I also want to express my gratitude to other philosophers: Sean Kelly, Tommie Shelby, and Alison Simmons, who each guided me through my journey as an undergraduate and graduate student at Harvard University. Besides them, Sally Haslanger at MIT and Kate Manne at Cornell University have championed my work.

Julie Tyler Ruiz, I am grateful for your teaching and encouragement as I learned the tools of creative writing. I would not have been able to write this book without your feedback and confidence in me. My critique group partners, Ellen Ellzey and Grace Santamaria, who saw parts of the first draft, also deserve special recognition. In addition, my Shut Up and Write! group has been an immense resource during the composition of this book. A hearty thank you goes to all the participants, particularly the old-timers—Marlene Bumgarner, Adrienne Cobb, Daniel Cohen, Darcé Costello, Jeanette Doherty, Annie Feldman, Marcie Geffner, Christine Hanlon, Michele Hathaway, Gale Johnson, Immy Kwuon, Smadar L., Gail Leinwall, Sarra Lev, Martin Lowry, A. T. Lynne, Joy Peltier, Evyn Rubin, Kim Smuga-Otto, and our founder, Lauren Sprang. I also want to recognize my co-hosts, who took turns with me to facilitate the group: Theresa Barker, Sherry Cornell, Marilyn Hartman, Diane O'Neill, Carol Park, and Cecilie Schulze.

My colleagues at Florida International University are the most welcoming group of philosophers I have met, and the undergraduate majors are the most passionate group of students I have had the privilege to teach. I thank you wholeheartedly for your trust in me. A special shoutout to all my students in Philosophy of Gender and Race, as well as Feminism and Philosophy, who shared their enthusiasm for my work on body image.

Several therapists cared for me during the trials of my graduate studies and career as a professor. More than anyone, I thank my eating disorder counselor, Dalit Szkolnik, for her support throughout the stages of my recovery. I'm indebted to you for your scrumptious recipes, savvy advice, and steadfast kindness. You saw me through two rounds of counseling and never lost faith in me.

Amanda Bernardi, you've been a wonderful agent. I am grateful for your determination as you pitched the book. Thank you, Jas Respess, my editor at North Atlantic Books, for helping me refine my ideas and complete the final draft. Sam Haselby at *Psyche* first assisted me in sharing the ideas in this book with a broad readership. Barry Lam and the 2024 cohort of the Marc Sanders Foundation Philosophy in Media Fellowship also shaped my approach to writing philosophy for a general audience. Gabriel Olano, a brilliant student at Christopher Columbus High School and now an undergraduate at Columbia University, provided tireless assistance on my Substack and kept me up to speed with Gen-Z trends. Many thanks to all of you for helping this book come into the world.

Since college, I've been blessed with the most loving friends anyone could wish for. Linnea Gandhi, you've been my cheerleader for over twenty years. Emily McWilliams and Elizabeth Miller, I love how we bonded over being the only women in our PhD cohort and mastered the challenges of graduate school. Dare I say that our camaraderie was a feminist practice? Annie Castro, our weekly walks and coffee dates have grounded me. Elizabeth Scarbrough, thank you for your generous comments on parts of the manuscript and unflagging support of my efforts as a writer. Your collegiality, companionship, and comfort have brightened my days on and off campus. Charles More, you introduced me to Steven Pressfield's ideas and taught me that Resistance was the enemy of my creativity. I hope that by writing this book, I've "turned pro." Thank you for your meticulous look over the entire manuscript and suggestions to help bring readers into the (philosophical) fold. I couldn't imagine reaching the finish line without you all.

A final and special thank you goes to my family. Mama, thank you for your virtual cooking lessons and for checking on my writing progress. Papa, ever the sportsman, thank you for teaching me to appreciate my body for all it can do. Pepita, thank you for your unending interest in my philosophical work. Archie, you're an amazing pup. Manue, thank you for being my funny and off-the-wall sister: You're a star! And so is your canine companion, Riley. Above all, thank you to my oh-so-special terrier, Carol, for dragging me on walks when I could only think of finishing my book, for being by my side when I was typing furiously in the final stretch, and for watching me read craft books at happy hour. You are the love of my life.

Index

C

About the Author

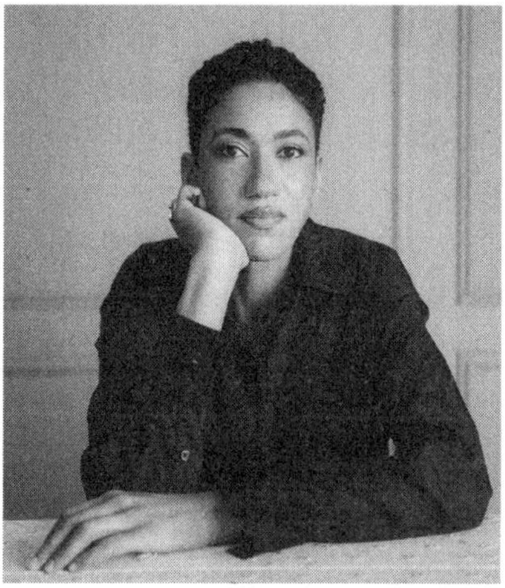

PHOTO BY JORGE ECHEVARRIA

Céline Leboeuf is an associate professor of philosophy and affiliate faculty in Women, Gender, and Sexuality Studies at Florida International University. In her research, she addresses questions about beauty and the body. How are standards about physical appearance shaped by gender and race? What does it feel like to be sexually objectified? Why can't we shake the pressure to shrink our bodies into sizes we can't sustain in the long term?

Her essays for a general audience have appeared in Substack, the *Project Vox* blog, and *Psyche*. She has been sought out for her expertise in publications such as *Vogue*, *The Atlantic*, and *The New York Times*, on topics ranging from body positivity to inclusivity in swimwear. This is her first book.

About North Atlantic Books

North Atlantic Books (NAB) is an independent, nonprofit publisher committed to a bold exploration of the relationships between mind, body, spirit, and nature. Founded in 1974, NAB aims to nurture a holistic view of the arts, sciences, humanities, and healing. To make a donation or to learn more about our books, authors, events, and newsletter, please visit www.northatlanticbooks.com.